Alternative Medicine
and
Multiple Sclerosis

Alternative Medicine and Multiple Sclerosis

Allen C. Bowling, M.D., Ph.D.

Associate Medical Director
The Rocky Mountain Multiple Sclerosis Center
Englewood, Colorado

and

Clinical Assistant Professor of Neurology
University of Colorado Health Sciences Center
Denver, Colorado

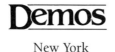

Demos

New York

Demos Medical Publishing Inc., 386 Park Avenue South, New York, New York 10016

Library of Congress Cataloging-in-Publication Data

Bowling, Allen C.
    Alternative medicine and multiple sclerosis / Allen C. Bowling.
        p. ; cm.
    Includes bibliographical references and index.
    ISBN 1-888799-52-8 (pbk.)
    1. Multiple sclerosis—Alternative treatment.
    (DNLM: 1. Multiple Sclerosis—therapy.   2. Alternative Medicine.   WL 360
B787a 2000)   I. Title.
    RC377 .B68 2000
    616.8'3406—dc21

                                                                00-064516

Made in the United States of America

Dedication

To my wife, Diana

Contents

Complementary and Alternative Medicine

Types of Therapy

Summary

References   235

Index   241

Foreword

The following is a common scenario presented to multiple sclerosis (MS) specialists by their patients on a daily basis:

"Doctor, I recently began treatment with these vitamin/mineral supplements, phytochemicals, herbs, and evening primrose oil at the recommendation of my cousin. A friend advised me to start treatment with magnets, and now I own magnetic inserts for my shoes and a magnetic mattress to sleep on. I am also adjusting my diet at the recommendation of my chiropractor, exercising regularly, attending hydrotherapy classes, practicing yoga, and considering chelation therapy. My mother wants me to start treatments to strengthen my immune system and have my dental amalgams removed. When I went to the pharmacist yesterday to pick up my MS medicine he recommended that I talk to you about these new and effective Procarin patches. What do you think about what I am doing for my MS? Do any of these treatments work in MS? Will they affect what you recommend to treat my MS?"

Before 1997, my common answer to a patient's attempts at self-directed care and integration with conventional medicine was a carefully crafted and intellectually honest, "I don't know." This was not a very satisfying answer for my patients and certainly did not acknowledge their sincere attempts to help themselves in dealing with an incurable disease. Our patients were attempting to do the right thing for their health but lacked the knowledge base to synthesize the recommendations being put before them. These recommendations come from a variety of sources and can be rather compelling to a person with MS, especially when accompanied by positive testimonials. In my discussions with other MS specialists, they had a similar paucity of knowledge from which to respond appropriately to their patients.

In early 1997, the staff and my colleagues at the Rocky Mountain Multiple Sclerosis Center surveyed our patients about their use of complementary and alternative medicine (CAM). We found that approximately two-thirds use some form of CAM and that most do so under their own initiative and guidance. The majority combine CAM with treatments recommended by their physicians. With this information in hand, it was time for us to become knowledgeable about CAM and begin giving our patients answers with substance.

Dr. Allen C. Bowling took up this tremendous and difficult challenge. He is uniquely trained, having earned his medical degree and Ph.D. degree in pharmacology from the Yale University School of Medicine. He then completed neurology training at the University of California–San Francisco and fellowship training at Massachusetts General Hospital and Harvard Medical School. He has done research in the areas of diet and the relevance of antioxidants to neurologic disease. Dr. Bowling has spent nearly three years researching CAM specifically as it applies to MS. Over the last two years, he has given numerous well-received seminars on CAM in MS to patients and health care providers. At the Rocky Mountain MS Center, we are seeing our patients respond favorably to the information presented by making rational decisions in integrating CAM with other treatments. We are now able to provide them with solid facts about new interventions they are trying or contemplating. This has strengthened our relationship with our patients.

With this authoritative book, people with MS as well as health care professionals can readily look up an intervention or treatment and find out the origins, merits, and available evidence for use in MS. The information in this book should help stimulate disease-specific research into CAM. We hope that the reader will find this information to be timely and useful.

Ronald S. Murray, M.D.
President and Medical Director
Rocky Mountain MS Center
Englewood, CO

Preface

This book was written to provide accurate and helpful information about complementary and alternative medicine (CAM) to people with multiple sclerosis (MS). The term CAM refers broadly to medical approaches, such as acupuncture or herbal medicine, that are not typical components of conventional medicine. Despite the fact that the majority of people with MS appear to use CAM, it is difficult to find reliable information about the relevance and usefulness of these therapies in MS. Those who practice a therapy or who are selling products may not understand MS or may exaggerate claims in order to make sales. On the other hand, physicians and other health care professionals often have little or no information or experience in CAM and may not have the resources to provide accurate information to their patients. It is hoped that this book will fill the current information gap in this area.

There are many potential benefits to providing CAM information. People with MS may realize that there are unconventional treatment options that may offer relief and hope for situations in which there are limited conventional medical therapies. Providing access to reliable CAM information should also allow people to avoid potentially dangerous interactions between CAM therapies and conventional medicine and to distinguish CAM therapies that are possibly effective, low risk, and inexpensive from those that are ineffective, dangerous, or costly. Finally, it is hoped that the objective information in this book will remove some of the prejudices and misperceptions that are rampant in this area, stimulate serious thought and discussion about CAM and MS, and lead to further study of those therapies that are widely used or appear promising.

This book is divided into three main sections. The first section provides a general introduction to MS and CAM. The second section, which is the main portion of the book, presents detailed information on a large number of CAM modalities. This section is organized alphabetically, which should allow the reader to quickly find information on a particular CAM therapy. The final section includes a chapter that organizes the information in a way that should allow people with specific symptoms to identify potentially useful CAM therapies. At the end of the book, there is a "Glossary of Popular Supplements," which is a quick source of MS-relevant information about commonly-used supplements.

A large number of references were used to write this book. More than 50 books and more than 2,000 scientific and clinical journal articles were reviewed. The most relevant books and journal articles are listed under "Additional Readings" at the end of the chapters. These readings include technical as well as nontechnical material. In addition, when specific data are mentioned in the text, a numerical reference is given that may be found in a detailed reference section at the end of the book. Most of the books that are referenced should be available through public libraries, medical libraries, or bookstores. Summaries or abstracts of the journal articles may be found by "Medline" searches, available through the website of the National Library of Medicine (www.nlm.nih.gov). The entire articles may be obtained from medical libraries.

Organization of Chapters and Reading Sequence

The second section of this book evaluates many different CAM therapies, which are arranged alphabetically so that they are easy to locate. This arrangement of chapters may be awkward if you intend to read through the entire book. A possibly useful organization and reading sequence is one based on the National Institutes of Health classification for CAM. If this sequence is followed, the structured reading sequence is as follows:

Biologically-Based Therapies

Diets—Diets and Fatty Acid Supplements
Herbal Medicine
    Herbs
    Marijuana
    Aromatherapy
Orthomolecular Medicine
    Vitamins, Minerals, and Other Nonherbal Supplements
Pharmacological, Biological, and Instrumental Interventions
    Allergies
    Aspartame
    Bee venom therapy
    Candida treatment
    Chelation therapy
    Cooling therapy
    Dental amalgam removal
    Enzyme therapy
    Hyperbaric oxygen
    Neuralyn
    Procarin
    Toxins

Alternative Medical Systems

Acupuncture and Traditional Chinese Medicine
Ayurveda
Homeopathy
T'ai Chi

Lifestyle and Disease Prevention

Exercise

Mind-Body Medicine

Biofeedback
Hypnosis and Guided Imagery
Meditation
Music Therapy
Pets
Prayer and Spirituality
Yoga

Manipulative and Body-Based Systems

Massage and Body Work
    Chiropractic medicine
    Craniosacral therapy
    Feldenkrais
    Massage
    Pilates Method
    Reflexology
    Tragerwork
Unconventional Physical Therapies
    Colon therapy
    Hippotherapy and Therapeutic Horseback Riding

Biofield Medicine

Therapeutic Touch

Bioelectromagnetics

Magnets and Electromagnetic Therapy

Acknowledgments

$\mathcal{M}$any individuals and organizations made this book possible. First, I would like to thank my wife, Diana, for her invaluable, unwavering support. She offered provocative insight into the subject, encouraged me during the challenging times, and helped create time for me to write. Also, I thank our two daughters, Elizabeth and Sarah, for tolerating my time away from home and for teaching me regularly that in daily life, as in medicine, there are many different perspectives on a given situation.

This book would not have been possible without the support of the Board of Directors and the staff at the Rocky Mountain MS Center. From the initial stages, Dr. Ronald Murray, President of the MS Center, encouraged the development of this project. Thomas Stewart, JD, PA-C, played a critical role by devoting time and energy to the research and by providing creative input and inspiration. Patricia Kennedy, RN, CNP, and Lee Shaughnessy read the manuscript carefully and made valuable suggestions. Lee Shaughnessy, Dr. Ragaa Ibrahim, and Julie Lawton assisted with the research. Linda Graham and Kathy Haruf helped type the manuscript.

Many of my patients at the MS Center motivated me to write this book. Through my patients, I learned that many were quite devoted to CAM therapies. I realized that I knew little about some of these therapies that obviously were an important component of their health care. I respect my patients for their willingness to openly share their feelings and experiences related to CAM, and I thank them for providing first-hand information that was critical in the development of this book.

A number of organizations and individuals provided valuable advice, information, and financial or moral support: Therese Beaudette, RD; my parents, Dr. Franklin Bowling and Ruth Bowling, RD; Scott Boynton, DiplAc, BAc; Dr. Jay Schneiders; Joan Wolk at Demos Medical Publishing; HealthONE Foundation; Denver Botanic Gardens; Hudson Gardens. Lastly, I thank Dr. Diana M. Schneider at Demos Medical Publishing for her ongoing support, thoughtful input, and openness to pursue this controversial subject.

Alternative Medicine
and
Multiple Sclerosis

Complementary and Alternative Medicine

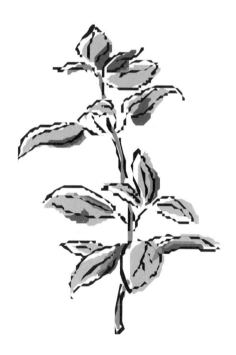

Introduction

$\mathcal{M}$ultiple sclerosis (MS) is a common disease of the nervous system. Most people with MS use some form of conventional medical treatment. In addition, many people also use complementary and alternative medicine (CAM), which refers to unconventional medical practices that are not part of mainstream medicine. Despite the fact that CAM is used frequently and MS is a common neurologic disorder, it is difficult to obtain accurate and unbiased information specific to the use of CAM for MS.

Before considering the relevance of *unconventional* medicine to MS, it is important to understand the approach of *conventional* medicine to this disease. There have been dramatic advances recently in the field of MS research. Through scientific studies, we now have an increased under-standing of the disease process itself. Also, clinical studies with experi-mental medications have yielded new therapies that slow the progression of MS and control MS-related symptoms, such as stiffness or pain.

Who Develops MS?

MS is a common neurologic disease that affects approximately 350,000 people in the United States. Women are diagnosed with the disease about twice as frequently as men. Although MS may affect people in all age groups, it is typically diagnosed between the ages of 20 and 40. There is a striking relationship between the prevalence of MS and the geographic area in which an individual lived during childhood. In general, an individual has a higher risk of developing MS if he or she grew up in an area that is far from the equator and a lower risk if the childhood years were spent near the equator.

How Does MS Affect the Nervous System?

In contrast to many diseases that affect a single part of the human body, MS affects two different body systems, the immune system and the nervous system. The *immune system* is not a distinct organ like the brain or liver. Instead, it is composed of many different types of molecules and cells (known as white blood cells) that travel through the blood stream. The immune cells use chemical messages to protect the body from attack by bacteria, viruses, and cancers. MS is an "autoimmune" condition in which the immune system is excessively active in such a way that it attacks the *nervous system*. The part of the nervous system that is involved in MS is the central nervous system (CNS), which includes the brain and spinal cord. The nerves in the CNS communicate with each other through long wire-like processes that have a central fiber (axon) surrounded by an insulating material (myelin). In MS, the immune system cells cause injury to the myelin. Recent studies indicate that there is damage to the axon as well. The injury to the nerve cells results in slowing or blocking of nerve impulses that prevents the affected parts of the nervous system from functioning normally.

The cause of MS is not entirely clear. It is believed that there are two important factors in developing the disease, one of which is environmental and the other is genetic. The environmental factor may be a virus that individuals are exposed to during childhood. This could relate to the characteristic increased prevalence of MS in areas distant from the equator; a specific viral infection of childhood could be more common in temperate climates distant from the equator.

The presence of a genetic factor is suggested by family studies that demonstrate a hereditary predisposition to MS. Some genetic diseases are "dominant" and are clearly passed down through generations. MS is usually not passed on in such a well-defined pattern. Rather, there may be an inherited *predisposition* to the disease that must be present in addition to an environmental agent.

What Symptoms Do People with MS Experience?

The symptoms of MS depend on which areas of the brain and spinal cord develop MS lesions. For example, if the nerve that is involved in vision (the optic nerve) develops a lesion, blurring of vision occurs. This is referred to as *optic neuritis*. If a lesion develops in the part of the brain that produces movement on the left side of the body, left-sided weakness develops. In addition to visual blurring and weakness, other common MS symptoms include fatigue, depression, urinary difficulties, walking unsteadiness, stiffness in the arms or legs, tingling, and numbness.

The time course over which MS lesions develop and the number and location of lesions is different for each individual. Consequently, the time frame in which symptoms occur and the specific types of symptoms experienced is unique for each person. Also, as a result of the large variability of lesions between individuals, MS varies greatly in severity. Some people may have rare, mild attacks over their lifetime and may not experience any permanent symptoms, while others may develop severe, permanent symptoms over a relatively short period of time.

MS symptoms may occur episodically or may progress continuously. Episodes of symptoms are known as relapses, attacks, or exacerbations. There usually is improvement in symptoms after an attack; this improvement is referred to as a "remission." In contrast to these "relapsing-remitting" symptoms, some people have symptoms that develop slowly and then progressively worsen over time with no clear remissions; these symptoms are referred to as "progressive."

Specific combinations of relapsing-remitting and progressive symptoms are the basis for classifying MS. People who experience attacks and then improve have "relapsing-remitting MS." This is the most common type of MS at the time of diagnosis. Some people who initially have relapsing-remitting disease may subsequently develop progressive symptoms; this is known as "secondary progressive MS." People who have progressive symptoms from the onset of the disease, which is relatively rare, have "primary-progressive MS." Individuals with "progressive-relapsing MS" have progressive symptoms from the onset, as occurs with primary progressive MS, but they also experience intermittent relapses.

Conventional Medical Therapy for MS

Dramatic advances have been made recently in the treatment of MS. In the past, there were no particularly effective therapies for changing the course of disease. Since 1993, three medications for MS have been approved by the U.S. Food and Drug Administration (FDA): interferon beta-1b (Betaseron®), interferon beta-1a (Avonex®), and glatiramer acetate (Copaxone®); a fourth drug, Rebif® (an interferon beta-1a), is available in Canada but not in the United States. These drugs decrease the number and severity of relapses, slow the progression of the disease, and decrease the development of new brain lesions.

Because of the positive effects of these medications, all people with MS should be strongly considered for treatment with one of these drugs. A 1998 statement by the National MS Society emphasized the importance of treatment. The statement recommended that treatment with these medications should be started soon after an MS diagnosis is made and should be considered in all people with MS, regardless of age, rate of relapses, and level of disability.

In addition to the beta interferons and glatiramer acetate, several other medications are used to treat MS. *Steroids* are used for exacerbations. These may be taken orally (prednisone, dexamethasone) or intravenously (methylprednisolone or Solumedrol®). Some chemotherapy medications, including methotrexate, azathioprine (Imuran®), and cyclophosphamide (Cytoxan®), are occasionally used to attempt to slow disease progression.

Given the wide range of symptoms caused by MS, there are multiple treatment possibilities. Therapies for symptoms include medications and nonmedication approaches, such as physical therapy, occupational therapy, speech therapy, and psychotherapy. Common MS symptoms that are treated with these therapies include fatigue, depression, weakness, incoordination, walking difficulties, stiffness, bowel and bladder disorders, and sexual difficulties.

For more information on conventional approaches to MS, the reader is referred to other more extensive texts in this area (see "Additional Readings" at the end of this chapter).

Complementary and Alternative Medicine

Complementary and alternative medicine (CAM) is a controversial area. In fact, even the term and its definition are not entirely agreed upon. Besides complementary and alternative medicine, other frequently used terms are *unconventional* medicine and *integrative* medicine. The term *complementary medicine* refers to therapies that are used *in addition to* conventional medicine, while the term *alternative medicine* is used to describe treatment that is used *instead of* conventional medicine.

There are many different definitions of CAM. These definitions frequently state what CAM "is not" as opposed to what it "is." For example, in the United States, CAM is sometimes defined as medical therapy that is not widely taught at American medical schools or is not generally available in American hospitals. This definition recently has become less clear because CAM is now part of the curricula of many medical schools and is provided more often in the medical community. Also, as clinical trials are done to evaluate the effectiveness of CAM therapies, some forms of CAM may eventually become components of conventional medicine.

CAM includes a vast number of therapies. Multiple schemes have been proposed for categorizing these diverse and often unrelated therapies. One classification scheme and some representative examples of therapies are:

- Biologically based therapies: diets, herbs, vitamins, other supplements, bee venom therapy, hyperbaric oxygen
- Alternative medical systems: acupuncture, Ayurveda, homeopathy
- Lifestyle and disease prevention: exercise
- Mind-body medicine: relaxation methods, biofeedback, t'ai chi, yoga
- Manipulative and body-based systems: chiropractic, massage, reflexology
- Biofield medicine: therapeutic touch
- Bioelectromagnetics: magnets, pulsing electromagnetic fields

Many studies have documented that CAM is used frequently in the United States. One well-known large study was conducted in 1997 and was reported in the medical literature in 1998 by Dr. David Eisenberg (1). In this study of more than 2,000 people, approximately 42 percent used some form of CAM. It was estimated that 629 million visits were made to practitioners of alternative medicine; this was greater than the number of visits to all primary care physicians in that year. Nearly 20 percent of people were taking some type of herb or vitamin along with a prescription medication. Most people used CAM without the supervision of a CAM practitioner, and most people did not discuss its use with their physician. As a result, nearly half of the people were using CAM without the advice of a physician or a CAM practitioner. This demonstrates the need for increased patient–physician communication in this area.

This 1997 study was a follow-up to a previous study conducted in 1990 (2). From 1990 to 1997, CAM use increased by 25 percent, and the yearly visits to CAM practitioners increased by 47 percent. Interestingly, there was *no* change in the percentage of people who did not discuss CAM use with their physicians; approximately 60 percent did not discuss CAM use with their physicians in both studies.

The 1990 and 1997 studies found a high use of CAM in people with chronic conditions such as MS. In addition, the 1997 study found that CAM use was relatively high in women and in people between the ages of 35 and 49; this sex and age distribution is similar to that of many people with MS. These findings suggest that CAM use may be more prevalent in people with MS than in the general population.

CAM Use in MS

Several studies have evaluated CAM use in MS. A large published study was conducted in Massachusetts and California in the 1990s (3). Approximately 60 percent of people had used CAM, and, on average, people used two to three different types of CAM. We conducted a similar survey in 1997 at the Rocky Mountain MS Center and found that approximately two-thirds of those who responded to the survey used CAM. These studies indicate that the majority, or approximately two-thirds, of people with MS use some form of CAM.

A different type of study, reported in 1999, examined visits to CAM practitioners by people with MS (4). This study did not evaluate overall CAM use, and, of note, most people who use CAM do not visit a practitioner. When CAM use in this study is compared with CAM use in the general population study of Dr. David Eisenberg, it appears that people with MS visit CAM practitioners about 40 percent more often than does the general population. Overall, these studies indicate that CAM use is higher in people with MS than in the general population.

In surveys of people with MS and of the general population, a consistent finding is that CAM is usually used in conjunction with conventional medical therapy. In other words, CAM is usually used in a *complementary* way. Approximately 90 percent of people who use CAM also use conventional medicine. This leaves a relatively small fraction of people who use CAM in a truly *alternative* manner.

It is sometimes erroneously believed that there are only two preference groups for medical therapy, one group that uses only conventional therapy only and another group that uses only CAM therapy. In fact, there is a third "mixed" group that combines conventional medicine and CAM. Importantly, the studies of CAM use in people with MS demonstrate not only that this "mixed" group exists but also that it actually appears to represent the majority.

With a large number of people with MS pursuing CAM therapies, it is essential for people to be knowledgeable about the therapies they choose and for physicians, other healthcare providers, and CAM practitioners to be aware that multiple conventional and CAM therapies are in use and that interactions among them are possible.

People with MS use a wide range of CAM therapies. Those that appear to be especially popular include massage, dietary supplements, diets, chiropractic medicine, acupuncture, meditation and guided imagery, and yoga. Reasons for people with MS to pursue CAM are as varied as the different CAM modalities used. In the Massachusetts and California survey

(3), the most common reason for choosing a particular CAM therapy was that a person had heard of another person benefiting from that therapy. Two other popular reasons were that mainstream medicine did not relieve symptoms or did not have a cure for the disease.

Information About CAM and MS

For CAM in general, the information available to the general public is vast but of variable quality. For CAM that is relevant to MS, the amount of information is limited and the quality is also variable. To attempt to understand the type of information that is available on CAM and MS, we conducted an informal survey of the popular literature on CAM at the Rocky Mountain MS Center. At two local bookstores, we found 50 CAM books written for a lay audience. Two-thirds of these books had sections on MS. In some books, MS was incorrectly defined as a form of muscular dystrophy. Other books made the erroneous—and potentially danger-ous—statement that, because MS is an immune disorder, it is important to take supplements that stimulate the immune system. In fact, MS is an immune disorder, but it is characterized by an *excessively active* immune system; thus, immune-stimulating supplements may actually be harmful. On average, the CAM books recommended five or six therapies for MS. In 20 percent of them, 10 or more therapies were recommended. It was rare for books to discourage the use of any CAM treatment. Interestingly, none had the same recommended therapies. In general, therapies that are used more frequently by patients appear to be those that are recommended more often in books; the fact that this information is full of inaccuracies is therefore troubling.

In addition to books, information about CAM can be obtained from vendors of products and CAM practitioners. Unfortunately, product ven-dors, such as people who sell supplements, often exaggerate claims about their products. Practitioners of CAM (as well as product vendors) some-times have limited experience with MS and are not certain how their ther-apy relates to such a specific and complex disease process.

Physicians and other mainstream healthcare providers are another potential source of information about CAM. Unfortunately, this group gen-erally is not trained or experienced in CAM use and, for a variety of rea-sons, often is reluctant to become involved in this area. Even for conven-tional healthcare providers who are interested in CAM, only limited objec-tive and accessible MS-specific information is currently available in the medical literature.

People with MS are "Caught in the Middle"

Many people with MS pursue some form of CAM but may not readily be able to obtain objective and practical information. They may seek out CAM books, products, or practitioners, but find that MS is not specifically addressed or that claims of the effectiveness of the therapy are exaggerated. On the other hand, they may attempt to obtain CAM information from their physician or other healthcare provider and find that little or no information is available. In this way, pursuing CAM can be frustrating and confusing for people with MS.

This book was written to provide objective MS-relevant CAM information to people with MS. Also, because the area of CAM is changing rapidly, we developed a website devoted to CAM and MS at the Rocky Mountain MS Center. This site, http://www.ms-cam.org/, is updated regularly and has interactive features. This site has several missions:

- To create a worldwide community of people interested in CAM and MS
- To provide accurate and unbiased information
- To allow users to discuss their experiences with CAM through threaded discussions
- To conduct surveys to assess the effectiveness and safety of CAM therapies for people with MS

A Matter of Perspective

CAM is controversial for many different reasons. One important issue to keep in mind is that of perspective. Because of the differences in perspective, mainstream healthcare providers and people with a disease may view the same set of facts differently.

Physicians view the use of basic science and rigorous clinical trial methods as a powerful tool to develop new disease understanding and new therapies. People with MS may believe that this process is powerful, but that it is also slow and may yield limited advances during their lives.

The "gold standard" for developing new therapies is known as a *randomized, controlled clinical trial*. This clinical testing employs specific and rigorous methods, including the use of a placebo-treated group, "blinding" of patients and investigators (such that neither patients nor investigators know who has received placebo and who has received active medication), and randomly selecting those who will receive placebo or active medication. Physicians and other mainstream healthcare providers generally use therapies only after they have been found to be effective in these well-designed clinical trials. Through this process, there is a black and white distinction between those therapies that have been proven effective in clinical trials and those that have not.

Some of the interest and controversy in CAM stems from the fact that there may not be such a black and white distinction but rather shades of gray. For example, some therapies have not undergone rigorous large-scale clinical testing, but scientific studies in animals or small clinical studies in people have produced promising results. These types of therapies are not generally incorporated into mainstream medicine. However, people with a disease may have an interest in such promising therapies, especially if they are relatively safe and inexpensive.

Another difference in patient–physician perspective is apparent with proven mainstream therapies. Conventional medications that are 30 to 40 percent effective may represent a major advance for physicians and other healthcare providers but, for people with MS these therapies may be seen as 60 to 70 percent away from a cure (which would be 100 percent effective).

In some areas of CAM, the same set of facts is viewed negatively by conventional medicine and positively by some people with MS. This emphasizes the importance of first establishing the facts about a therapy and then realizing that these facts may be interpreted differently by mainstream healthcare providers and people with MS. Under some circumstances, it is as if there are two different cultures, that of the healthcare provider and that of the person who has the disease, and these two cultures may have strikingly different belief systems.

The difference in perspective becomes especially apparent when a physician develops a disease. In this situation, there may be a dramatic shift in an individual's attitudes about what constitutes an appropriate medical therapy. There have been several published examples of this shift in perspective.

Dr. Alexander Burnfield, an English psychiatrist who has MS, wrote a book entitled *Multiple Sclerosis: A Personal Exploration*. With reference to evening primrose oil, he states: "I started taking it before the research was published and, being only human, take it just in case I get worse if I stop. This is, I know, an unscientific and emotional response, and the logical-doctor part of me is quite shocked" (5).

Dr. Elizabeth Forsythe, also an English physician with MS, wrote *Multiple Sclerosis: Exploring Sickness and Health*. With reference to diet and MS, she states: "It is what you feel in your own body and mind that is the most important thing and it is very easy for doctors and patients to forget that. I believe that a little of what you fancy does do you good!" (6).

In *Healing Lessons*, Dr. Sidney Winawer, chief of gastroenterology at Memorial–Sloan Kettering Hospital in New York City, gives a provocative account of his transformational experiences with CAM through his relationship with his wife, who pursues various unconventional and unproven cancer therapies. He writes: "I failed to see that Andrea's cancer, of all things, would wake us up. I knew least of all that my beliefs as a doctor were about to be turned upside down" (7). He also begins to view therapies from a different perspective: "I shared her conviction that uncertain hope was better than hopeless certainty" (8).

A Unified Perspective

Should we abandon these mainstream methods because basic science research has not fully elucidated the cause of MS and clinical trials have not developed a cure? NO. These methods of conventional medicine provide the greatest hope for understanding and curing MS. The difficulty is that MS is a complex disease, and an uncertain amount of future work is needed.

Should we acknowledge that there are areas of CAM that may be of interest to people with MS because conventional medicine does not have a cure for MS? YES. It is a disservice to people with MS who have an interest in CAM to not acknowledge that these therapies exist. Part of this acknowledgment should involve providing accurate information. By focusing more attention on CAM, we may actually develop a new understanding of the disease process and perhaps discover new therapies.

It is possible to simultaneously acknowledge, respect, and use conventional medical therapy and CAM therapy. This dual approach is a way to bring together the sometimes disparate views of mainstream healthcare providers and people with MS.

Additional Readings

Books

Burnfield A. *Multiple Sclerosis: A Personal Exploration*. London: Souvenir Press, 1997.

Cassileth BR. *The Alternative Medicine Handbook*. New York: W.W. Norton, 1998.

Dillard J, Ziporyn T. *Alternative Medicine for Dummies*. Foster City, CA: IDG Books, 1998.

Forsythe E. *Multiple Sclerosis: Exploring Sickness and Health*. London: Faber and Faber, 1988.

Fugh-Berman A. *Alternative Medicine: What Works*. Baltimore: Williams & Wilkins, 1997.

Kalb RC. *Multiple Sclerosis: The Questions You Have—The Answers You Need.* 2nd ed. New York: Demos Medical Publishing, 2000.

Schapiro RT. *Symptom Management in Multiple Sclerosis.* 3rd ed. New York: Demos Medical Publishing, 1998.

Spencer JW, Jacobs JJ. *Complementary/Alternative Medicine: An Evidence-Based Approach.* St. Louis: Mosby, 1999.

Winawer SJ. *Healing Lessons.* Boston: Little, Brown, 1998.

Journal Articles

Berkman CS, Pignotti MG, Cavallo PF, et al. Use of alternative treatments by people with multiple sclerosis. *Neurorehab Neural Repair* 1999; 13:243–254.

Eisenberg D, Davis R, Ettner S, et al. Trends in alternative medicine use in the United States, 1990–1997. *JAMA* 1998; 280:1569–1575.

Eisenberg D, Kessler R, Foster C, et al. Unconventional medicine in the United States. *N Engl J Med.*1993; 328:246–252.

Schwartz C, Laitin E, Brotman S, et al. Utilization of unconventional treatments by persons with MS: Is it alternative or complementary? *Neurology* 1999; 52:626–629.

Placebos and
Psychoneuroimmunology

When considering any type of medicine, whether unconventional or conventional, it is important to understand and recognize the significance of placebos and the placebo effect. The beneficial effects of placebos highlight the complexity of treating human disease and are necessary to consider when evaluating the effects of any therapy.

Placebos and the Placebo Effect

A *placebo* is generally thought of as a "dummy pill" or "sugar pill." More formally, a placebo is a therapy that is not believed to have a specific effect on the disease or the condition for which it is given. "Placebo" is derived from Latin and means "I will please." A placebo may be given in the form of a substance or a procedure. The *placebo effect* is a response of a person's condition to the placebo.

There are many dramatic examples of the placebo effect. One of the early examples in medical literature involved a woman with excessive nausea and vomiting during pregnancy. She was told she was being given a medication for nausea but was actually given syrup of ipecac, which is known to induce vomiting and is sometimes given to children who have swallowed a possibly toxic substance. The woman in this study actually had *improvement* in her nausea.

A well-known study of the placebo effect was reported in 1955 by Dr. Harry Beecher (1). He described the placebo effect in a variety of conditions, including the common cold, pain after surgery, headache, and seasickness. Overall, symptoms were improved in 35 percent of the people who were given the placebo. Subsequent studies of a variety of medical conditions found placebo effects that were frequently in the range of 30 to 40 percent. In some studies, placebos have been 70 percent effective.

As would be expected, a placebo effect occurs in studies of people with MS. A notable response to placebos has been observed in studies of therapy for MS itself as well as for MS-related symptoms. In older MS studies from 1935 to 1950, a variety of ineffective therapies produced 60 to 70 percent improvement. More recently, trials with chemotherapy drugs in MS showed a placebo effect on the rate of MS attacks. In recent research studies with interferon beta-1b (Betaseron®), the first FDA-approved immune therapy for MS, the number of MS attacks was determined for people taking Betaseron and for another group taking placebo. The placebo-treated group had a 28 percent decrease in the rate of MS attacks. Similarly, the placebo group showed decreased attack rates of 33 percent in trials with interferon beta-1a (Avonex®) and 43 percent in trials with glatiramer acetate (Copaxone®). In all of these trials, the study drug was *significantly more effective than the placebo*, and this finding is the basis for the widespread use of these medications.

There are several explanations for the decrease in MS attack rates observed with placebos. This may represent the natural course of the disease or it may be an artifact of statistics (referred to as "regression to the mean"), but it may also represent a genuine placebo effect.

Placebo responses have also occurred in studies that use biological tests to monitor disease activity. Magnetic resonance imaging (MRI) is frequently used in MS clinical trials. A recent MRI study of a small number of people with MS found that the placebo-treated group had an approximately 20 percent reduction in the development of new brain lesions (2). This finding was not statistically significant, but this may have been due to the small number of people in the study.

A particularly interesting finding occurred in a study of an experimental medication, alpha-interferon (3). People with MS were given alpha-interferon or placebo. They were evaluated by determining the rate of attacks. Both the treated group and the placebo group had a 60 to 70 percent decline in the rate of MS attacks. The investigators also measured the activity of an immune cell known as a *natural killer cell*. The natural killer cell activity was evaluated because it is known that its activity is increased by alpha-interferon. As expected, the group treated with alpha-interferon showed a 52 percent increase in natural killer cell activity. Surprisingly, the placebo group showed an increase in natural killer cell activity that was nearly identical to that of the alpha-interferon group.

Placebo effects have been observed in other MS clinical studies, including those that have evaluated treatment for symptoms caused by the disease. For MS-associated fatigue, the placebo effect in clinical trials has been as high as 50 percent.

These studies suggest that there may be a powerful influence of the mind over a disease process such as MS as well as over the activity of the immune system.

Interaction of the Nervous System and the Immune System

In the past, there was thought to be little interaction between the nervous system and the immune system. However, recent studies demonstrate that there *are* ways in which the nervous system and the immune system communicate with each other. The placebo effects observed in people with MS and other diseases may be examples of this process. The field of study that examines immune system–nervous system interactions has been termed "psychoneuroimmunology."

There are many different ways by which the brain may communicate with the immune system. The brain influences the production of hormones, which then may affect the function of the immune system. In addition, nerve fibers have connections with immune organs. The chemical messengers used by the nervous and immune systems appear to be involved in cross-communication. Nerve cells communicate with each other by releasing chemicals known as *neurotransmitters*, while immune cells communicate with each other by secreting different chemicals known as *cytokines*. Research studies have shown that cytokines may influence nerve cell activity and that neurotransmitters may influence immune cell function. Thus, the nervous system and the immune system do not appear to function independently but rather are components of a network in which they communicate and alter each others' activity.

Because there appear to be important interactions between the nervous system and the immune system, modifying brain activity may alter the immune system and immune diseases such as MS. For example, psychological stress and depression may influence the functioning of the immune system. One way to manage stress is to write about stressful life events. The act of writing about such events has been associated recently with improved immune function and improvement in two immune diseases, rheumatoid arthritis and asthma.

A variety of studies have evaluated the influence of the nervous system on MS activity. In animals, injury to one component of the peripheral nerves (nerves that are outside the brain and spinal cord), the sympathetic nervous system, leads to altered immune function and worsening of experimental allergic encephalomyelitis (EAE), an animal model of MS.

Many studies have examined the possible influence of psychological stress on MS. At this time, the effect of stress on MS is not clear. Two research studies indicate that the period three to six months before an MS attack is associated with stressful life events. Other studies, however, have not shown a clear association between stress and MS.

Placebos and CAM

Placebos and the placebo effect are important when considering conventional and unconventional medicine. In conventional medicine, the placebo effect is often disregarded or minimized. In clinical trials of experimental drugs, the placebo response is simply subtracted from the effect of the drug. Also, there is a certain level of discomfort for placebos within conventional medicine. Dr. Jay Katz states: "... if placebos were to be acknowledged as effective in their own right, it would expose large gaps in medicine's and in doctors' knowledge about underlying mechanisms of care and relief from suffering" (4).

For studies of MS, which is an extremely individualized, variable, and unpredictable disease, it is clear that any evaluated therapy must be compared with a placebo. Sometimes CAM therapies are touted on the basis of the experience of individuals; these are known as "anecdotes." Because of the placebo effect and the fact that MS may remain stable with no therapy or that full recovery may occur after an MS attack, it is important not to rely heavily on treatment benefits based only on anecdotes. Whether a therapy is conventional or unconventional, definitive claims of effectiveness must be based on studies of large numbers of people, some of whom are treated with placebos.

Finally, an important difference between conventional medicine and CAM may relate to the placebo effect. It has been stated that much of the history of medicine is actually the history of the placebo effect because medicine has not, until recently, had particularly effective therapies. Physicians in the past may have relied very heavily on establishing relationships with patients and may have become skilled at administering ineffective therapies in a way that maximized the placebo response.

Modern mainstream medicine has undergone significant changes. It has become more technological. Much of medicine is now focused on the body alone instead of on the body and the mind. Decreased insurance reimbursement has led to briefer physician visits. With all of these changes, many physicians lack the resources and time to nurture strong patient relationships and to develop optimal methods for administering therapies. In contrast to the past history of medicine, the recent history of some aspects of American medicine may be the history of *removing* the placebo effect from clinical practice.

In contrast to physicians, many practitioners of CAM probably spend more time with patients and rely more on positive interpersonal skills to interact with and treat them. This may be true for practitioners in areas such as acupuncture, homeopathy, and massage. A single session with these practitioners may last 60 minutes or longer and involve detailed discussion of many topics, while physician visits are often 10 to 20 minutes or shorter and focus exclusively on diseases, symptoms, diagnostic tests, and drug therapies. Regardless of the effectiveness of their therapies, some practitioners of CAM may be more skilled and more comfortable than physicians with using the power of the placebo effect.

Additional Readings

Books

Brody H. *The Placebo Response*. New York: HarperCollins, 2000.
Harrington A, (ed.). *The Placebo Effect: An Interdisciplinary Exploration.* Cambridge: Harvard University Press, 1997.
Shapiro AK, Shapiro E. *The Powerful Placebo*. Baltimore: Johns Hopkins University Press, 1997.

Journal Articles

Chelmicka-Schorr E, Arnason BG. Nervous system–immune system interactions and their role in multiple sclerosis. *Ann Neurol* 1994; 36:S29–S32.
Hellemans A, Enserink M. Can the placebo be the cure? *Science* 1999; 284:238–240.
Hirsch RL, Johnson KP, Camenga DL. The placebo effect during a double blind trial of recombinant alpha2 interferon in multiple sclerosis patients: immunological and clinical findings. *Neuroscience* 1988; 39:189–196.
La Mantia L, Eoli M, Salmaggi A, et al. Does a placebo-effect exist in clinical trials on multiple sclerosis? Review of the literature. *Ital J Neurol Sci* 1996; 17:135–139.

Important Precautions About Complementary and Alternative Medicine and MS

This book provides much detailed information about specific types of CAM. This information is intended to assist people in assessing CAM therapies for MS. In addition to this specific information, there are some general ideas that are important and may be helpful in the CAM decision-making process.

■ *The information in this book should not be used to be "converted" to CAM and should not be taken as a recommendation to use specific types of CAM.*

Conclusive evidence about the effectiveness and safety of most forms of CAM is not available. Consequently, this book provides information but does not make recommendations. Because this book does not specifically promote the use of CAM, it is hoped that individuals who are not interested in CAM will not feel any need for "conversion" to it. For those individuals who are already interested in CAM, the information in this book should be helpful in assessing the possible effectiveness, safety, and cost of different therapies. Without specific recommendations, the way in which the information is used and the decision about whether to pursue CAM therapy rests with the individual. Ultimately, individuals must decide on their own about using CAM, and they must assume the risks and responsibilities of pursuing a specific CAM therapy.

■ *Be aware of when it is reasonable to pursue CAM.*

It is reasonable to consider CAM therapy in some situations. For example, it would be reasonable to consider CAM for a symptom that is of low intensity, such as mild muscle stiffness or mild pain. CAM also may be worth pursuing for a condition in which conventional medical therapy is ineffective or only partially effective. Forms of CAM to consider are those that are possibly effective, are probably safe, are of low–moderate cost, and require only a reasonable amount of effort.

On the other hand, severe symptoms, such as prominent muscle stiffness or excruciating pain, or a serious disease process such as MS, should not be treated *solely* with CAM. In these situations, it may be reasonable to pursue CAM in addition to conventional therapy. In other words, using CAM in a complementary way may be appropriate. CAM therapy should not be pursued if there is little or no reliable information about effectiveness, safety, or cost. Therapies to avoid are those that are probably ineffective or unsafe or involve high expense or great effort.

■   *Have a plan about using CAM.*
Several steps need to be taken when using any form of CAM:

- ■   Consider conventional medicine first.
- ■   Evaluate and address the reason(s) for wanting to use CAM.
- ■   Obtain accurate information about effectiveness, safety, cost, and the effort involved.
- ■   If CAM is chosen, *discuss it with your physician*, monitor your response, and discontinue the treatment when appropriate.

■   *Use caution.*
It is important to include a physician in this process because most CAM practitioners do not have a physician's broad knowledge base about the diagnosis and treatment of medical conditions.

■   *Realize that information about most forms of CAM is incomplete.*
Many forms of conventional medical therapy have undergone rigorous testing of effectiveness and safety. In contrast, data are limited for most CAM therapies, especially in terms of specialized studies of people with MS or studies of the effects of therapies on immune system activity. As a result, it is often only possible to make a "best guess" about the effectiveness and safety of CAM. As more studies are done on CAM, some of these "best guesses" may be found to be incorrect. For example, a therapy that is currently thought to be "possibly effective" or "probably safe" may conceivably be found with further studies to be definitely ineffective or definitely unsafe. Thus, there is a certain amount of risk involved in pursuing CAM.

In terms of slowing down the MS disease process, there is no "magic cure." No forms of CAM therapy have undergone sophisticated clinical testing similar to that of glatiramer acetate (Copaxone®), interferon beta-1b

(Betaseron®), and interferon beta-1a (Avonex® and Rebif®). As a result, these therapies should be considered by all people with MS before pursuing CAM.

■ *Be aware of the "telltale signs" of unreliable forms of CAM.*
Several features often indicate that a CAM therapy has not been well studied, is provided by an unreliable source, or is being promoted with exaggerated claims. Some of these "telltale signs" are:

■ Heavy reliance on testimonials—the benefits of a therapy are sometimes reported in accounts known as testimonials, which may not be entirely accurate and which describe the treatment response of a single person as opposed to that of a large, well-studied group of people.

■ Strong claims about effectiveness—terms such as "amazing" and "miraculous"—should raise suspicions; if it sounds too good to be true, it probably is.

■ A single therapy is claimed to be an effective therapy for many different medical conditions.

■ The composition of a therapy is "secret."

■ Little or no objective information is available on effectiveness, safety, or cost.

■ Therapy involves inpatient treatment, injections, or intravenous medication.

■ There is an antiscience or anticonventional medicine attitude—this may be conveyed through claims of "conspiracies" or through an unwillingness of a CAM practitioner to work cooperatively with a physician.

■ *Recognize that MS is a disease that involves excessive immune system activity.*
In some lay books on CAM, MS is described as an immune disorder, and it is then assumed that therapies that stimulate the immune system should be beneficial for MS. Some books may even recommend 5 to 10 supplements that activate the immune system. Using this faulty reasoning, therapies that are recommended for MS are sometimes the same as those recommended for acquired immunodeficiency syndrome (AIDS) and cancer. Also, the vague term *immunomodulator* is sometimes used to describe supplements that appear to stimulate the immune system.

This approach and these recommendations are inaccurate and potentially dangerous. Although MS is, indeed, an immune disorder, it generally involves *too much*, not too little, immune system activity. Consequently, CAM therapies that increase the activity of the immune system could worsen the disease process. In contrast to MS, AIDS and cancer may benefit from treatment that activates the immune system. Thus, in general, immune-stimulating therapies that may be helpful for AIDS and cancer may actually be harmful for MS.

■ *Do not confuse scientific evidence with clinical evidence.*

Potential MS therapies may be evaluated scientifically through "test tube" experiments or by using an animal model of MS known as experimental allergic encephalomyelitis (EAE). The most important (and most expensive and laborious) test of a therapy, however, is to give it to people with MS and to carefully monitor their response. It is essential to realize that scientific studies are imperfect and that therapies that are promising in scientific experiments are not necessarily clinically effective therapies for people with MS. There is a long list of experimental compounds that are effective in suppressing the immune system or treating EAE but are ineffective for treating people with MS. There are even some therapies (for example, interferon gamma, lenercept, and antibodies to tumor necrosis factor) that are effective in treating animal models of MS but actually worsen disease in people with MS.

■ *Avoid misconceptions about supplements.*

Many misconceptions are sometimes promoted by vendors of supplements. These misconceptions include:

■ Compounds are sometimes claimed to be safe and beneficial if they are "natural"—while some natural compounds are safe and beneficial, some are toxic (for example, deadly chemicals that are present in mushrooms and many other plants), and many are not effective therapies for any disorder.

■ Some supplements, especially herbs, are claimed to have beneficial effects and no side effects—supplements (like prescription medications) that have beneficial effects must contain chemicals that may also potentially produce side effects.

■ More is not necessarily better—it is sometimes believed that the use of high doses of a single supplement or a large number of different supplements is more beneficial than the use of low doses or a single supplement; however, in most cases, supplements in high doses or large numbers are probably not more effective and may, in fact, be more likely to produce side effects.

■ Combinations of supplements with conventional medications have not been fully investigated—supplements are sometimes taken in addition to conventional medications (for example, evening primrose oil and one of the FDA-approved injectable MS medications); the effectiveness and safety of these "combination therapies" has not been investigated; notably, there are some situations in which combination therapy is less effective or more likely to produce side effects than single-treatment therapy.

The precautions discussed in this chapter have been incorporated into the discussions in this book. These rules should be helpful for evaluating CAM therapies not mentioned here or for assessing CAM therapies for conditions other than MS.

Types of Therapy

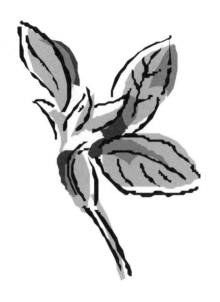

Acupuncture and Traditional Chinese Medicine

$\mathcal{A}$cupuncture is one of many components of what is known as traditional Chinese medicine, a healing method that has been in use for more than 2,000 years. Traditional Chinese medicine is now used by approximately one-fourth of the world's population. In Western countries, the use of traditional Chinese medicine, especially acupuncture, has grown over the past two decades. It is now estimated that more than one million Americans are treated with acupuncture yearly.

The recognition of acupuncture by Western medicine is not entirely new. In the late 1800s, Sir William Osler, one of the most honored and respected physicians and medical educators, wrote a textbook of medicine in which he recommended acupuncture for low back pain and sciatica. In 1901, *Gray's Anatomy*, a classic medical text, also referred to acupuncture as a treatment for sciatica.

There are five components of traditional Chinese medicine. In addition to acupuncture, they include traditional Chinese herbs, diet and nutrition, exercise, stress reduction and counseling, and massage. T'ai chi, which is discussed elsewhere in this book, is also a component of traditional Chinese medicine. This chapter discusses acupuncture as well as two types of herbal medicine, Asian herbal medicine and Asian proprietary (or patent) medicine.

Acupuncture

Acupuncture is based on a complex theory of body functioning that is very different from the Western biological approach. Briefly, it is believed that there is a free flow of energy or "qi" through 14 main pathways or "meridians" on the body. There is also a balance of opposites known as "yin" and "yang." Disease is believed to result from a disruption in the normal flow of this energy.

Treatment Method

Acupuncture involves the insertion of thin, solid, metallic needles into specific points on the meridians. It is believed that this alters the flow of energy and thereby produces improvement. There are approximately 400 acupuncture points. Fortunately, not all of these are used in a single session! Four to 12 points are typically used in a session.

For those wary of needles, methods other than needle insertion may be used to stimulate acupuncture points. The application of finger pressure to these points is known as *acupressure* or, in Japan, *shiatsu*. Small hot cups are placed on points with *cupping*, and electrically stimulated needles are used with *electroacupuncture*. Transcutaneous electrical nerve stimulation (TENS) is a variant of electroacupuncture that is sometimes used. In *moxibustion*, smoldering fibers of an herb, Asian mugwort or "moxa," are placed on acupuncture points or are used to heat needles that are then placed in acupuncture points.

How could a needle stuck into the skin possibly provide pain relief and other medical benefits? Many answers to this question have been proposed. One explanation for the pain-relieving effects of acupuncture is that it releases "opioids," chemicals produced by the body that decrease pain. In preliminary studies using a special type of magnetic resonance imaging (MRI), acupuncture at pain-relieving acupuncture sites produced changes in brain activity. These changes, some of which occurred in pain-relevant brain regions, were present during the time in which the pain-relieving effects were also present. Acupuncture may alter the levels of other chemical messengers in the body, decrease stress, or simply act as a placebo. In the end, it may be found that multiple processes are involved.

Studies in MS and Other Conditions

A large number of studies have evaluated the effectiveness of acupuncture. Unfortunately, many of these studies have been small and not well conducted. To attempt to understand the possible medical benefits of acupuncture, the National Institutes of Health (NIH) organized a 12-member panel in 1997 to review the studies on acupuncture (1). The panel concluded that there was "clear evidence" for acupuncture being effective for nausea and vomiting associated with surgery, chemotherapy, and possibly pregnancy. Evidence for effectiveness was also found for pain after dental procedures and several other types of pain. The report concluded that "the data in support of acupuncture are as strong as those for many accepted Western medical therapies" and that acupuncture was a "reasonable option" for some conditions.

It is surprising how few studies have evaluated acupuncture in MS. A Canadian study of eight people with MS in 1974 showed that a few had some mild and brief benefits (2). However, there did not appear to be long-lasting effects. A very small study of two people with MS in 1986 showed that multiple MS symptoms improved (3).

A recent survey evaluated acupuncture use in 217 people with MS in British Columbia (4). The preliminary results of this survey indicate that approximately two-thirds reported beneficial effects. Many symptoms were improved, including pain, spasticity, bowel and bladder difficulties, tingling, weakness, walking difficulties, incoordination, and sleep disorders. The few side effects that were reported were pain and soreness at the needle site and a worsening of some symptoms (fatigue, spasticity, dizziness, and walking unsteadiness). One person associated acupuncture with provoking an MS attack. Overall, the results of this survey are promising. It must be kept in mind, however, that this was a self-assessment survey, not a formal clinical trial.

A 1986 study of 28 people with MS evaluated responses to stimulation at acupuncture sites (5). Interestingly, acupuncture sites were more sensitive in people with MS, and needle insertion provoked stiffness and muscle spasms. These findings may simply reflect a generalized MS-associated skin hypersensitivity or a tendency to muscle stiffness.

Some studies have evaluated the effectiveness of acupuncture for symptoms that may occur with MS. In these studies, however, the underlying disease was not MS. Limited studies suggest beneficial effects of acupuncture for weakness in people with strokes. In studies of variable quality, it has been found that acupuncture may be effective for other symptoms that may occur with MS, including anxiety, depression, pain (including facial pain, low back pain, and neck pain), dizziness, and urinary difficulties.

An important issue for MS is whether acupuncture has an effect on the immune system. At this time, the impact of acupuncture on immune system activity is not well understood. Although no studies have been done specifically in people with MS, acupuncture studies on immune system activity have been done in people with various forms of cancer and rheumatoid arthritis. Acupuncture has been associated with stimulating, inhibiting, and having no effect on the immune system. Because of these mixed results, further studies are needed to clarify this area.

Given the probable benefits of acupuncture in other medical conditions, it would be reasonable to pursue detailed studies of its effects in MS. Rigorous studies of the effect of acupuncture on the course of the disease would be expensive and difficult. In contrast, it would be feasible to evaluate the effects of acupuncture on some MS-associated symptoms, including pain, spasticity, weakness, and urinary disorders. If acupuncture were found to be effective for symptoms, it could be a useful therapy. However, treatment of chronic symptoms might need to be long-term, which may not be practical.

Side Effects

In general, acupuncture is a well-tolerated procedure, especially when done by a well-trained acupuncturist. The NIH panel that evaluated acupuncture stated: "the occurrence of adverse events . . . has been documented to be extremely low"(1). The panel also concluded that acupuncture was "remarkably safe with fewer side effects than many well-established therapies."

Over a 20-year period, only 216 serious acupuncture-related complications were reported worldwide. Serious complications are often caused by poorly trained or negligent acupuncturists. For people with MS, it is important to realize that acupuncture may produce drowsiness in up to one-third of people. This effect could conceivably be worse in people who have MS-associated fatigue or in those who take potentially sedating medication such as lioresal (Baclofen®), tizanidine (Zanaflex®), or diazepam (Valium®).

There are other rare acupuncture-associated risks. Sterile disposable needles should be used to avoid hepatitis and AIDS. People with damaged or prosthetic heart valves should probably not be treated with acupuncture because of the risk of infection. People who take blood-thinning medication (warfarin or Coumadin™) may occasionally experience bruising or, more rarely, bleeding complications. Electroacupuncture may produce heart rhythm abnormalities in people with a pacemaker, and the fumes from moxibustion may worsen breathing in people with asthma. These and other precautions of acupuncture are shown in Table 1.

TABLE 1. *Precautions with Acupuncture Use*

Avoid with:	Blood-thinning medication (warfarin or Coumadin™)
	Damaged or prosthetic heart valves
	Pacemaker (electroacupuncture)
Use caution with:	Immune-suppressing drugs or conditions
	First trimester of pregnancy
	Metal allergy
	Acupuncture sites in thorax (risk of lung or heart injury)

Practical Information

Acupuncture is usually done once or twice weekly. Sessions typically cost $45 to $60. The length of time required for a course of treatment varies. If a beneficial response occurs, it should usually be noted after 6 to 10 sessions. The length of a complete course of treatment depends on the specific symptoms and the underlying disease process. A longer treatment course may be necessary for MS and other chronic diseases.

In the United States, there are approximately 10,000 licensed acupuncturists, 3,000 of whom have M.D. or D.O. training. Organizations that can be helpful in obtaining information about acupuncture and locating an acupuncturist include:

- American Association of Acupuncture and Oriental Medicine (www.aaom.org), 433 Front Street, Catasauqua, Pennsylvania 18032 (610-266-1433)
- American Certification Commission for Acupuncture and Oriental Medicine (www.nccaom.org) 11 Canal Center Plaza, Suite 300, Alexandria, Virginia 22314 (703-548-9004)
- A listing of physicians or osteopaths who have acupuncture training is available from the American Academy of Medical Acupuncture (800-521-2262)

Conclusion

Acupuncture is usually well tolerated, but there are rare adverse effects. Variable results have been obtained in studies of MS and acupuncture. In small and preliminary studies, MS-associated symptoms that have responded to acupuncture are anxiety, depression, dizziness, pain (including facial pain, low back pain, and neck pain), bladder difficulties, and weakness.

Asian Proprietary Medicine (or Asian Patent Medicine)

Asian proprietary medicine, also known as Asian patent medicine, is a form of Asian herbal medicine. Preparations of this type of medicine usually contain mixtures of herbs as well as animal parts and minerals.

Several studies of the chemical composition of these preparations have found that they frequently contain potentially toxic ingredients. Recent data indicates that approximately one-third of these products contain drugs or dangerous metals. Drugs that have been found include diazepam (Valium®), steroids, and prescription asthma medications. Toxic metals sometimes found in these products are arsenic, mercury, lead, and cadmium.

Because of the possible presence of these toxic ingredients, Asian proprietary medicine should be avoided or used with extreme caution.

Asian Herbal Medicine

Asian herbal medicine involves therapy with herbal preparations that are often complex mixtures of many different herbs. Asian herbal medicine is frequently used in combination with acupuncture, but it may also be used on its own. There are several different ways in which Asian herbal medicine may be administered, including tablets, pills, powders, capsules, or tinctures. Raw herbs or extracts of herbs may also be used.

When considering the use of Asian herbal medicine, it is essential to know which specific herbs are being used and to recognize that the full range of effectiveness and toxicity has not been fully established for any of these herbal preparations. These issues and other important factors related to herbal medicine in general are discussed in more detail in the section on herbs. In addition, the section on herbs has information on some Asian herbs, including Asian ginseng, astragalus, dong-quai, ephedra (ma huang), and licorice. (See "Herbs.")

Studies in MS and Other Conditions

There is limited information about Asian herbal medicine in the treatment of MS. Several studies have been reported, but they are difficult to interpret because most of them have been published in Chinese and only summaries are readily available in English (6). One Chinese study in 1990 reported beneficial effects with herbal treatment in 35 people with MS. Another study reported by the same research group in 1995 found that Ping Fu Tang, a mixture of 17 different herbs, decreased the rate of MS attacks. There are several other MS studies of Chinese herbal medicine as well as Japanese herbal medicine. Paradoxically, in one of these studies, an herb that appears to stimulate the immune system, *Ganoderma lucidum*, was reported to slow the disease course in five people with MS. Overall, because these studies are not available in English, it is impossible to rigorously evaluate them or to make any clear conclusions about the research results.

Several specific Chinese herbs suppress the activity of the immune system and therefore could be therapeutic for MS. These herbs include Re Du Qing, Berberis, and *Tripterygium wilfordii*. Of these herbs, the most extensively studied is *Tripterygium wilfordii*, also known as Thunder God Vine, three-wingnut, or lei-gong-teng. Scientific studies indicate that this herb decreases the activity of T cells and other specific components of the immune system. In addition, it lessens the severity of experimental allergic encephalomyelitis (EAE), an animal model of MS. One study conducted in China with ten people with MS found that *Tripterygium wilfordii* produced "significant" improvement in eight people and mild improvement in two people.

Tripterygium wilfordii has been studied primarily in autoimmune disorders other than MS. Beneficial effects have been noted in animals with an experimental form of lupus. Some clinical improvement has been noted in people with rheumatoid arthritis and lupus.

At this time, studies are too limited for this therapy to be recommended specifically for MS or other autoimmune conditions. In addition, use of this herb has been associated with serious side effects (see below).

Side Effects

If considering Asian herbal medicine, people with MS should be aware of individual herbs or herbal mixtures that may stimulate the immune system (Table 2). The immune-stimulating effects of these herbs have been shown in scientific tests or in laboratory animals. Their effects on humans in general or on people with MS have not been specifically investigated. Thus, the immune-stimulating activity of the herbs represents a theoretical risk for people with MS.

"Fu-zheng" therapy, a type of Chinese herbal medicine, is believed to improve the ability of the body to defend itself. The two herbs used in Fu-zheng therapy, astragalus and *Ligustrum lucidum*, have been shown to activate immune

TABLE 2. *Asian Herbal Medicine That May Stimulate the Immune System*

Chinese:	Asian ginseng	Japanese:	Kakkan-to
	Acanthopanax obovatus		Kanzo-bushi-to
	Angelica sinensis		Shosaiko-to
	Artemis myriantha		
	Artemisia annua		
	Astragalus		
	Coix		
	Ge-gen-tang		
	Green tea		
	Licorice		
	Ligustrum lucidum		
	Reishi mushroom		
	Salvia miltiorrhiza		
	Shiitake mushroom		
	Sophora flavescens		
	Xiao-chai-hu-tang		

cells. Licorice and Asian ginseng, which are present in many different types of Chinese herbal medicine, have diverse effects on the immune system, including stimulating activities. Green tea contains potent antioxidant compounds, which may also produce immune-stimulating activity; this is discussed elsewhere in this book (see "Coffee and Other Caffeine-Containing Herbs").

Some types of Japanese herbal medicine have immune-stimulating properties (Table 2). Some of these mixtures are also used in Chinese medicine; for example, the Japanese herbs kakkan-to and shosaiko-to are the same as the Chinese herbs ge-gen-tang and xiao-chai-hu-tang, respectively.

Toxic effects have been associated with the use of some types of Asian herbal medicine (Table 3); they are not specific to MS. These herbs should be used with caution. Serious toxic effects on multiple body organs have been associated with some of these herbs. *Tripterygium wilfordii* has caused stomach upset, infertility, and on one occasion, death. Less significant tox-

TABLE 3. *Potentially Toxic Asian Herbs*

Aristocholia fangchi	Guiji
Baijiaolian	Jin bu yuan
Bushi	Licorice
Caowu	Ma huang (ephedra)
Chuanwa	Naoyanghua
Datura preparations	*Tripterygium wilfordii*
Fuzi	Yangjinhua
Guangfangji	

icity has been observed with the regular use of licorice, which may produce high blood pressure and low blood levels of potassium. The use of ma huang, or ephedra, has been associated with increased blood pressure, other dangerous side effects, and—rarely—death.

Practical Information

Chinese herbal medicine should be obtained from a trained herbalist. Monthly costs are approximately $20 to $60.

Conclusion

The use of Asian herbal medicine, especially on a long-term basis, should be considered with caution by people with MS. Reports of treatment benefits with this therapy cannot be fully evaluated because of the lack of published information in English. Some herbs may be toxic or may stimulate the immune system. The safety of long-term treatment has not generally been established.

Additional Readings

Books

Filshie J, White A. *Medical Acupuncture/A Western Scientific Approach*. Edinburgh: Churchill Livingstone, 1998.

Fugh-Berman A. *Alternative Medicine: What Works*. Baltimore: Williams & Wilkins, 1997, pp. 21–35.

Journal Articles

Borchers AT, Hackman RM, Keen CL, et al. Complementary medicine: A review of immunomodulatory effects of Chinese herbal medicines. *Am J Clin Nutrition* 1997; 66:1303–1312.

Chan TYK, Critchley JAJH. Usage and adverse effects of Chinese herbal medicines. *Human Exp Toxicol* 1996; 15:5-12.

Chan TYK, Chan JCN, Tomlinson B, et al. Chinese herbal medicines revisited: A Hong Kong perspective. *Lancet* 1993; 342:1532–1534.

NIH Consensus Development Panel on Acupuncture. *JAMA* 1998; 280:1518–1524.

Zhang L-H, Huang Y, Wang L-W, et al. Several compounds from Chinese traditional and herbal medicine as immunomodulators. *Phytother Res* 1995; 9:315–322.

Allergies

There is a long history of MS being associated with allergies. This idea was especially popular in the 1940s and 1950s. Many different allergic substances have been proposed over the years.

Various food allergies have been implicated in MS. Some studies have found that MS is more common in areas with high intakes of dairy products or gluten-containing grains, such as wheat, rye, oats, and barley. As a result, consumption of dairy products or gluten has been implicated in MS. Other proposed allergic foods have included yeast, mushrooms and other fungi, fermented products (such as vinegar), sugar, potatoes, red meat, fruits, vegetables, caffeine, and tea and other tannin-containing foods.

Treatment Method

There are several approaches to the treatment of allergies. If the allergic substance is a food, specific foods can be avoided. Another approach involves injecting the allergic substance under the skin; this leads to "desensitization," which decreases the response to the allergic agent.

Studies in Multiple Sclerosis

A limited number of studies have evaluated the possible role of allergies in MS. No well-designed studies exist to support any specific food or environmental factor as an allergic cause of MS. In addition, no studies have demonstrated that eliminating exposure to a certain presumed allergic agent is beneficial.

One suspected allergic substance that has been investigated is *gluten*, a protein that is present in wheat and wheat products. No benefit was found in a study of people with MS who did not consume gluten. Also, studies of the intestinal lining and blood have not demonstrated a sensitivity to gluten in people with MS.

It is interesting to note that people with MS actually appear to have *fewer* allergic problems than those who do not have the disease. Recent information indicates that people with MS have nearly 70 percent fewer allergic symptoms and more than 80 percent fewer positive allergy tests than the general population. This appears to be a result of the underlying immune disorder that occurs in MS.

Conclusion

At this time, there is no strong evidence to suggest that MS is associated with an allergic response to a specific food or environmental factor. Based on a limited number of studies conducted in this area, there is no reason to believe that allergy-free diets or desensitization procedures are beneficial for MS.

Additional Readings

Journal Articles

Hunter AL, Rees BW, Jones LT. Gluten antibodies in patients with multiple sclerosis. *Human Nutr-Appl Nutr* 1984; 38:142–143.

Jones PE, Pallis C, Peters TJ. Morphological and biochemical findings in jejunal biopsies from patients with multiple sclerosis. *J Neurol Psych* 1979; 42:402–406.

Tang L, Benjaponpitak S, DeKruyff RH, et al. Reduced prevalence of allergic disease in patients with multiple sclerosis is associated with enhanced IL-12 production. *J Allergy Clin Immunol* 1998; 102:428–435.

Aromatherapy

Aromatherapy is a type of healing that uses aromatic substances derived from plants. It was used in some form in ancient Egypt and ancient China. The type of aromatherapy that is currently used in the United States was originally developed in the early twentieth century by René Gattefosse, a French chemist.

Treatment Method

Aromatherapy is based primarily on the use of *essential oils*. These oils, which are of high quality and purity, are obtained from plants by a specialized distillation process or by cold pressing. More than 40 different essential oils are used. They may be used individually or as mixtures, and they are administered by direct application to the skin, mixing with bath water, or inhalation. Oils are sometimes applied to the skin by massage. In France, oils are sometimes taken internally by mouth or by the vagina or rectum. However, in general, oils should not be taken internally.

Like the other senses, the sense of smell serves an important role. Specific odors may trigger feelings and memories. Some studies have shown that certain odors may produce headaches or elicit relaxation. The nerve signals from the nose are transmitted to a part of the brain known as the *limbic system*, which is involved in emotion and motivation.

While smell is often thought of as a "minor" sense in humans, it is actually the major sense for many animals. For these animals, chemicals known as *pheromones* are detected by the olfactory system and are important for mating and communication.

Although the sense of smell is important and olfactory signals are sent to a brain region involved in basic psychological processes, the mechanism by which administering certain odors may be therapeutic is not clear.

Studies in MS and Other Conditions

Aromatherapy has not been systematically studied in people with MS. Studies of olfaction in MS indicate that 10 to 20 percent of people with the disease have an impaired sense of smell.

There are only a limited number of studies of the effects of aromatherapy on any medical condition, and those that do exist are generally of low quality. Many of the therapeutic claims about aromatherapy are based on tradition, not on actual clinical research.

Symptoms of MS that have been investigated in some aromatherapy research are anxiety, depression, and pain. For anxiety, studies of variable quality indicate that beneficial effects may be obtained with the use of lavender oil, Roman chamomile oil, and neroli (orange) oil. However, no large, well-designed clinical studies have examined this antianxiety effect. Preliminary information suggests that a lower dose of antidepressant medication may be needed by depressed men when the medication is used in combination with aromatherapy with a citrus fragrance. Lavender in bath water does not appear to relieve childbirth-associated pain.

Aromatherapy has been studied in a few other unrelated conditions. Small studies on older people with dementia have produced mixed results. Inhalation of black pepper extract may decrease the craving for cigarettes. People with a form of baldness called alopecia areata may benefit from scalp massage with a mixture of thyme, rosemary, lavender, and cedarwood oils.

When aromatherapy is combined with massage, as is often the case, it may be difficult to distinguish the benefits of the oil from those of the massage. In limited studies, massage alone has been associated with several beneficial effects, discussed elsewhere in this book, including alleviation of anxiety, depression, muscle stiffness, low back pain, and other types of pain.

Side Effects

Aromatherapy is usually well tolerated, but it is not risk-free. When applied to the skin, some oils may produce a skin rash (this type of allergic reaction may be detected by applying a small amount of oil to the skin and monitoring for a response for 24 hours). Approximately 5 percent of people appear to be allergic to fragrances. Because of possible toxic effects, oil should not be taken internally by mouth or any other method (this is especially true for eucalyptus, hyssop, mugwort, thuja, pennyroyal, sage, and wormwood). Pregnant women should probably avoid aromatherapy because the use of some oils may lead to miscarriage. If aromatherapy is combined with massage, the possible side effects of massage should be kept in mind (see also "Massage").

Practical Information

Aromatherapy may be obtained from a practitioner or may be self-administered. It is sometimes combined with herbal medicine or traditional Chinese medicine. A typical aromatherapy treatment session lasts 30 minutes.

More information on aromatherapy and aromatherapists may be obtained from:

- American Alliance of Aromatherapy, P.O. Box 750428, Petaluma, California 94975, 707-778-6762
- National Association of Holistic Aromatherapy, P.O. Box 17622, Boulder, Colorado 80308, 800-566-6735 or 303-258-3791

Conclusion

Aromatherapy is of low risk and reasonable cost. The benefits of this therapy in people with MS have not been systematically studied. Several small clinical studies suggest beneficial effects for anxiety and depression, but further research is needed. One large study found that aromatherapy was not effective for pain.

Additional Readings

Books

Dillard J, Ziporyn T. *Alternative Medicine for Dummies.* Foster City, CA: IDG Books, 1998, pp. 239–244.

Fugh-Berman A. *Alternative Medicine: What Works.* Baltimore: Williams & Wilkins, 1997, pp. 182–187.

Vickers A. *Massage and Aromatherapy: A Guide for Health Professionals.* London: Chapman & Hall, 1996.

$\mathcal{A}$spartame

$\mathcal{T}$here are some claims that aspartame, an artificial sweetener used in soft drinks, causes MS or worsens MS-associated symptoms.

Treatment Method

It is sometimes recommended that people with MS avoid all drinks and foods that contain aspartame.

Studies in MS and Other Conditions

No definitive studies have shown aspartame to cause MS or to worsen its symptoms. Limited studies indicate that it could provoke migraine headaches and worsen depression. In terms of other neurologic disorders, clinical studies do not indicate that aspartame worsens Parkinson's disease or epilepsy.

Aspartame is of potential concern because the body may convert aspartame to methanol and then convert the methanol to formic acid, which may produce serious toxicity. However, consuming moderate or even large quantities of diet soft drinks does not significantly increase blood levels of methanol or formic acid.

Conclusion

Given the results that are available at this time, there is no compelling reason for people with MS to avoid aspartame. There is no evidence that a reasonable intake of aspartame worsens MS or provokes MS-associated symptoms.

Additional Readings

Journal Articles

Leon AS, Hunninghake DB, Bell C, et al. Safety of long-term doses of aspartame. *Arch Int Med* 1989; 149:2318–2324.

Lipton RB, Newman LC, Cohen JS, et al. Aspartame as a dietary trigger of headache. *Headache* 1989; 29:90–92.

Van dewn Eeden SK, Koepsell TD, Longstreth WT Jr, et al. Aspartame ingestion and headaches: A randomized crossover trial. *Neurology* 1994; 44:1787–1793.

Walton RG, Hudak R, Green-Waite RJ. Adverse reactions to aspartame: double-blind challenge in patients from a vulnerable population. *Biol Psych* 1993; 34:13–17.

Ayurveda

Ayurveda was developed in India thousands of years ago and is the oldest known medical system still in use. Ayurveda means "knowledge (or science) of life" in Sanskrit, and its practice includes medicine and science as well as philosophy and religion. The form of Ayurvedic medicine that is now practiced is a modified version of the ancient form of this healing method. Ayurveda is still widely practiced in India. It has been popularized and promoted in the United States by Maharishi Mahesh Yogi and Dr. Deepak Chopra.

In Ayurveda, a harmonious relationship between mind, body, and spiritual awareness is believed to be important. The function of these entities is regulated by three physiologic principles known as "doshas." Disease is claimed to be the result of an imbalance of the doshas, and treatment aims to restore dosha balance. Like traditional Chinese medicine, Ayurveda holds that there is an important life force, called "prana."

Treatment Method

There are several components of Ayurveda. Like traditional Chinese medicine, pulse and tongue evaluation are important for diagnosis. Diet, exercise, lifestyle changes, and specific supplements are used therapeutically. Yoga, breathing exercises, massage, and meditation, discussed elsewhere in this book, are also components of Ayurveda. One type of Ayurvedic meditation, transcendental meditation (TM), was popularized by Maharishi Mahesh Yogi. Another important aspect of Ayurveda, "panchakarma," is used for disease prevention. Panchakarma means "five processes" and includes massages, sweat baths, vomiting, enemas, and bloodletting (through the use of leeches).

There are two primary types of Ayurveda outside India. Maharishi Ayur-Veda was started by Maharishi Mahesh Yogi and relies heavily on meditation. The other Ayurvedic school, advocated by Dr. Deepak Chopra, uses meditation in conjunction with other Ayurvedic methods.

Studies in MS and Other Conditions

No large published clinical studies have specifically investigated the effect of Ayurveda on MS or its symptoms. Some components of Ayurveda have been investigated individually. These include massage, meditation, and yoga, all of which are discussed in this book. These therapies may be helpful for some symptoms that occur with MS, including spasticity, pain, depression, and anxiety.

Some research has evaluated Ayurvedic supplements for other conditions. One small study found that the herb *Phyllanthus* was an effective therapy for liver inflammation; subsequent studies did not find beneficial effects. For asthma, mixed results have been obtained with an Ayurvedic preparation, *Tylophora indica asthmatica*. In experimental animal models of breast and lung cancer, beneficial effects have been shown for Maharishi-4, also known as Maharishi Amrit Kalash-4 or MAK-4. Curcumin, MA-631, and Maharishi-5, produce biochemical effects that might be beneficial for heart disease.

Side Effects

Ayurveda should not be used in place of conventional medicine for treating MS. Some Ayurvedic preparations contain dangerous metals, such as lead and mercury. These preparations have been associated with serious metal poisoning and should be avoided, even if they are claimed to be "deactivated" by heat.

Scientific studies indicate that some Ayurvedic supplements influence the immune system. Immune-stimulating activity has been noted in isolated scientific studies of Maharishi-4, Maharishi-5, *Boerhavia diffusa*, *Phyllanthus emblica*, and *Nimba arishta*. These preparations could theoretically be harmful to people with MS; clinical studies are needed to determine if they are in fact dangerous.

Ayurvedic remedies containing *Heliotropium* species have been associated with liver toxicity, which in some cases has led to death. Chemicals that may produce liver or kidney toxicity have been found in several Ayurvedic herbs, including *Cassia auriculata*, *Crotolaria juncea*, *Crotolaria verrucosa*, and *Holorrhena antidysenterica*. Kidney or liver toxicity in animals has been associated with *Aegle marmelos*, *Hemidesmus indicus*, *Terminalis chebula*, and *Withania somnifera*.

Practical Information

There is no program for licensing Ayurvedic practitioners in the United States. Ayurveda is practiced by a variety of healthcare professionals, including physicians, chiropractors, and nutritionists. Initial visits with Ayurvedic practitioners last approximately one hour; follow-up visits are briefer. The initial evaluation costs approximately $100 to $150 and usually is not covered by insurance. More information about Ayurveda and Ayurvedic medical practices may be obtained from local libraries and health food stores. Associations that provide information include:

- The American Association of Ayurvedic Sciences, 21151 12th Avenue NE, Bellevue, Washington 98004, 425-453-8022
- Ayurvedic Institute, 11311 Menaul NE, Suite A, Albuquerque, New Mexico 87112, 505-291-9698

Conclusion

Ayurveda is a healing system with relatively low risk and moderate cost. One component of Ayurveda, the use of specific supplements, may produce serious side effects and has not been fully studied in any medical condition, including MS. Other components of Ayurvedic practice, including massage, meditation, and yoga, may provide beneficial effects for anxiety, depression, pain, and spasticity.

Additional Readings

Books

Dillard J, Ziporyn T. *Alternative Medicine for Dummies*. Foster City, CA: IDG Books, 1998, pp. 109–118.

Fugh-Berman A. *Alternative Medicine: What Works*. Baltimore: Williams & Wilkins, 1997, pp. 36–38.

Spencer JW, Jacobs JJ. *Complementary/Alternative Medicine: An Evidence-Based Approach*. St. Louis: Mosby, 1999, pp. 75, 102, 140, 172.

Bee Venom Therapy and Other Forms of Apitherapy

Bee venom therapy, which is used by some people with MS, is one type of "apitherapy." This term refers to the use of bees or bee products to treat medical conditions. It is estimated that 5,000 to 10,000 people with MS in the United States use bee venom therapy.

Apitherapy has been used for thousands of years. It was used in ancient Egypt. Hippocrates used bee venom to treat arthritis in ancient Greece. Bee venom therapy has been used by famous leaders, including Charlemagne, Ivan the Terrible, and Charles the Great.

In more recent times, apitherapy, especially bee venom therapy, has been recommended by some people for MS and other autoimmune conditions, such as rheumatoid arthritis, lupus, and scleroderma. In the United States, Charles Mraz, also known as "The Bee Man," first advocated bee venom therapy in the 1930s. He initially treated his own arthritis effectively with bee venom therapy and subsequently recommended the treatment to people with arthritis and other inflammatory conditions, including MS. He claimed that the bee sting produces inflammation at the site of the sting and that the body then mounts an anti-inflammatory response. This anti-inflammatory response is believed to act not only against the sting but also against other inflammatory processes in the body.

Another popular recent advocate of bee venom therapy is Pat Wagner, known as "The Bee Lady." She has MS and claims to have used bee venom therapy effectively to treat herself.

Bee Venom Therapy

A variety of insects, collectively referred to as "bees," may inject venom through a burning sting. Honeybees are generally used for bee venom therapy. Along with wasps, yellow jackets, and hornets, honeybees are species in a family of insects known as Hymenoptera.

The venom of bees is produced by specialized cells. It has two purposes: to defend against attackers and to weaken or paralyze prey. Bee venom contains a mixture of substances. The pain and swelling that result from a bee sting are produced by chemicals, including histamine, dopamine, norepinephrine, and serotonin. Bee venom also contains several toxins that are known as apamin, melittin, mast-cell degranulating peptide, and minimine. Finally, bee venom contains proteins that are involved in allergic responses. These proteins (including phospholipase A2 and hyaluronidase) activate some immune cells and stimulate the production of one specific type of antibody, immunoglobulin E.

Bee venom contains many different substances. At this time, it is not known exactly how each of these substances interacts with the body and what effect they might have on a disease process such as MS.

Treatment Method

In bee venom therapy, a bee is usually grasped with tweezers and put on a particular part of the body. Tweezers are then used to remove the stinger 10 to 15 minutes after the sting. Ice is sometimes used on the skin before and after the sting to decrease the pain. Bee venom therapy typically is done in three sessions each week, and 20 to 40 stings are done in each session.

Studies in MS and Other Conditions

To attempt to determine the effect of bee venom on MS, studies have been done with experimental allergic encephalomyelitis (EAE), an animal form of MS. In these studies, mice with EAE were injected with honeybee venom three times weekly (1). Each injection was equivalent to 4 to 160 bee stings. Treatment with venom produced no benefit. In fact, in some animals, venom treatment may have produced worsening relative to those that received a placebo.

In this animal model of MS, further studies may evaluate whether one specific component of the venom may be more beneficial than the venom as a whole. Apamin, a chemical constituent of the venom, has some properties that could be beneficial for MS. Apamin inhibits the action of a component of the nerve cell known as the potassium channel. This is the same part of the nerve cell that is affected by the experimental drug 4AP (4-aminopyridine), which may be beneficial for MS-associated fatigue. However, it is not clear that bee venom therapy produces high enough levels of apamin in the central nervous system to significantly inhibit potassium channels. Further studies are needed in this area.

In terms of human studies of bee venom therapy in MS, there is no adequate information. There are isolated accounts of individuals with MS who improved after this treatment. However, no large-scale studies have yet evaluated its effectiveness in MS. In October 1999, a one-year study of the safety of bee venom therapy in humans began at Georgetown University. This safety study may be followed by a study of the effectiveness of bee venom therapy for MS.

Side Effects

As noted, bee venom therapy may worsen EAE, an animal form of MS. This indicates that it is possible that bee venom therapy could actually worsen MS.

In general, bee venom therapy is well tolerated. Death is a very rare, but obviously important, adverse effect. Approximately 40 cases of bee sting deaths occur annually in the United States. Bee sting deaths are frequently attributed entirely to severe allergic reactions ("anaphylaxis"), but many of these deaths actually may be due to heart attacks that occur as a result of the stress of a mild allergic reaction in combination with heat, dehydration, or underlying heart disease. Importantly, severe allergic reactions may occur in individuals who have no past history of reactions to bee stings. Because of the possibility of a severe allergic reaction, a bee sting kit should be available if bee venom therapy is used.

Another rare side effect of bee venom therapy that people with MS should be aware of is optic neuritis. This condition involves inflammation of the nerve that connects the eye to the brain. Optic neuritis may produce mild or severe impairment of vision and is one of the more common conditions produced by MS. There have been reports of stings on or near the eye producing an MS-like form of optic neuritis in people who do not have MS. It is sometimes recommended that bee stings be given to the temple or eyebrows for visual problems. It would be safest for people with MS (and people without MS) to *avoid bee stings in this area* because of the possibility of bee sting–induced optic neuritis.

Finally, it is important to note that no formal studies have evaluated the long-term safety of bee venom therapy. As a result, it is not known if chronic bee venom therapy use is associated with significant toxic effects that have yet to be identified.

Other Bee Products

A variety of bee products other than bee venom are also used in apitherapy. These products are often recommended for MS and symptoms that may occur with the disease, such as fatigue, weakness, visual difficulties, and memory problems. There is no evidence that these products are effective for MS or MS-associated symptoms.

Bee Pollen

Bee pollen, which is composed of plant pollens, plant nectars, and bee saliva, is sometimes recommended to lessen fatigue, increase strength, and improve many other ailments. It contains a variety of nutrients, but it may also be contaminated with rodent debris, bacteria, insects, and the eggs and feces of insects. There are rare reports of severe allergic reactions and worsened asthma after bee pollen use. Studies of bee pollen use in college and high school athletes have not demonstrated improvement in physical performance. There are no clear reasons for consuming bee pollen because it has no clear therapeutic properties and may have adverse effects.

Propolis

Propolis, a waxlike material that is also known as "bee glue," is collected by bees from buds on poplar and conifer trees and is used to repair cracks in hives. It may be weakly effective in killing a variety of bacteria and viruses. Limited studies have shown both stimulation and suppression of immune system activity. Propolis may facilitate the healing of mouth lesions. It has no other demonstrated health benefits. No studies have examined the safety of its use.

Raw Honey

It is sometimes claimed that honey contains valuable minerals and vitamins. Actually, honey contains approximately 80 percent sugar and 20 percent water. The mineral and vitamin content of honey is very low. Honey consumption is generally safe, but it has no clear therapeutic effects.

Royal Jelly

Royal jelly is recommended for many conditions, including some MS-associated symptoms such as weakness, depression, cognitive difficulties, and sexual problems. Royal jelly is a white substance that is produced by worker bees and is important in the development of queen bees. It has many chemical constituents, including neopterin, which is a compound secreted by immune system cells, and royalisin, a protein that has antibiotic activity. As with propolis, a small number of studies suggest that royal jelly may activate or suppress the immune system. Royal jelly may provoke asthma; in one case, royal jelly was associated with a fatal asthma attack. Royal jelly use has also been associated with allergic reactions, including nasal congestion, itching, hives, and severe breathing difficulties (anaphylaxis). People with asthma or significant allergies should use royal jelly with caution.

Practical Information

Anyone considering bee venom therapy should first discuss it with a physician. For possible allergic reactions, it is important to have a bee sting kit available and to know how to use it. The names of local beekeepers can be obtained from the U.S. Department of Agriculture. Other bee products are available in pharmacies, health food stores, and apitherapy specialty stores.

Conclusion

There are no well-documented benefits of bee venom therapy and other bee products for people with MS. In addition, this type of treatment produces rare, but potentially serious, adverse effects, which include severe allergic reactions and death with bee venom therapy, and allergic reactions and worsening of asthma with the use of other bee products.

Additional Readings

Books

Cassileth BR. *The Alternative Medicine Handbook*. New York: W.W. Norton, 1998:155–158.

Journal Articles

Lublin FD, Oshinsky RJ, Perreault, M, et al. Effect of honey bee venom on EAE. *Neurology* 1998; 50:A424.

Song H-S, Wray SH. Bee sting optic neuritis. *J Clin Neuro-opth* 1991; 11:45–49.

Biofeedback

Biofeedback uses the mind–body connection for therapeutic purposes. Biofeedback involves the use of machines to monitor bodily functions such as heart rate, pulse, or muscle tension. An individual undergoing biofeedback attempts to consciously alter one of these presumably "involuntary" bodily processes. The use of biofeedback has been investigated for many medical conditions.

Treatment Method

In biofeedback, monitoring equipment is used to translate the activity of specific bodily functions into images or sounds. The images may be seen on a computer screen or the sounds may be heard. The monitoring methods that are used depend on which physiologic activity is of interest: electromyography (EMG) biofeedback is used to monitor muscle tension; thermal biofeedback for skin temperature; electrodermal response for perspiration; respiration biofeedback for rate, rhythm, and volume of breathing; finger pulse biofeedback for pulse rate; and brainwave biofeedback for brain electrical activity.

In a biofeedback session, a biofeedback therapist assists an individual in altering the activity of a particular body process through mental or physical exercises. The individual learns methods to produce the desired change through feedback from the monitor, input from the therapist, and experimentation. These methods can eventually be used without the use of monitoring equipment.

Studies in MS and Other Conditions

Biofeedback may have applications for MS-related symptoms. For anxiety and insomnia, which may be significant problems in MS, biofeedback may be beneficial by promoting relaxation. It may also be helpful in treating some types of pain, although the use of biofeedback to treat MS-associated pain has not been formally studied.

Some research suggests that biofeedback may be helpful for people with urinary incontinence, a problem that may occur in MS. Medications and pelvic exercises are available for incontinence. These approaches may not be fully effective, however, and the medications may have undesirable side effects. Studies for biofeedback treatment of urinary incontinence have been reported with mixed results. Biofeedback may be especially effective for people who have difficulty knowing which muscles to contract with pelvic exercises. Studies need to be done to more fully evaluate biofeedback therapy for urinary incontinence, specifically for MS-related urinary incontinence.

People with MS may also experience incontinence of stool. Biofeedback may be beneficial for this problem. In people with stool incontinence related to conditions other than MS, biofeedback produces improvement in approximately 70 percent.

Finally, MS may produce *spasticity*, or stiffness in the arms and legs. Some studies in people with cerebral palsy indicate that spasticity may respond to biofeedback, but no large studies specifically with MS-associated spasticity have been done.

An interesting issue is whether biofeedback may be used to regulate the immune system and, conceivably, thereby alter immune diseases such as MS. Variable effects of biofeedback-induced relaxation on immune function have been obtained; no consistent results have been reported.

Biofeedback may be an effective treatment for many other conditions. Among neurologic disorders, people with strokes or with migraine or muscle-tension headaches may benefit. Also, biofeedback may improve circulation, mildly decrease blood pressure, and be beneficial for alcoholism, drug abuse, and posttraumatic stress disorder.

Side Effects

Biofeedback usually is very well tolerated. With electrodermal biofeedback, people with heart conditions and pacemakers should be cautious and should discuss the treatment with their physician.

Practical Information

Biofeedback should be obtained from a trained therapist. There are devices that can be self-operated, but biofeedback monitoring is a complex process that is most likely to be helpful when it is performed by a qualified practitioner. Biofeedback sessions typically last 30 to 60 minutes. The number of sessions required ranges from a few to 30 or 40. Health insurance sometimes provides coverage for this therapy.

Many trained biofeedback therapists are psychologists. Certification is provided by the Biofeedback Certification Institute of America. Biofeedback practitioners can be found in the telephone directory under psychologists or by obtaining a directory of biofeedback therapists from the Biofeedback Certification Institute of America (10200 West 44th Avenue, Suite 304, Wheat Ridge, Colorado 80033, 303-420-2902).

Conclusion

Biofeedback is a low-risk, moderate-cost therapy that may be beneficial for some MS-associated conditions. It may be especially helpful in situations in which conventional medical approaches are not fully effective or produce side effects. MS symptoms that may be responsive to biofeedback include anxiety, insomnia, pain, urinary incontinence, fecal incontinence, and muscle stiffness. Further studies are needed to fully evaluate the effectiveness of biofeedback for MS symptoms.

Additional Readings

Books

Cassileth BR. *The Alternative Medicine Handbook*. New York: W.W. Norton, 1998, pp. 117–121.
Fugh-Berman A. *Alternative Medicine: What Works*. Baltimore: Williams & Wilkins, 1997, pp. 41–46.

Journal Articles

Berghmans, LCM, Hendriks HJM, Hay-Smith EJ, et al. Conservative treatment of stress urinary incontinence in women: A systematic review of randomized clinical trials. *Br J Urol* 1998; 82:181–191.
de Kruif YP, van Wegen Erwin EH. Pelvic floor muscle exercise therapy with myofeedback for women with stress urinary incontinence: A meta-analysis. *Physiotherapy* 1996; 82:107–113.
Norton, C, Hosker, G, Brazzelli, M. Biofeedback and/or sphincter exercises for the treatment of faecal incontinence in adults (Cochrane review). In: The Cochrane Library, Issue 2, 2000. Oxford: Update Software.

Candida Treatment

$\mathcal{M}$S has been associated with infections with *Candida*, a species of yeast. The most common type of *Candida* is *Candida albicans*. Mild infections with *Candida* may involve the mouth, which is referred to as thrush, or the vagina, which is referred to as monilia. More significant infections with *Candida* usually occur in people with conditions that suppress the immune system, such as AIDS, and the use of chemotherapy medications. These infections may involve the mouth, throat, eye, heart, and blood stream.

It has been proposed that many medical conditions are associated with "overgrowth" of *Candida*, which is known as "Candidiasis hypersensitivity," "polysystemic candidiasis," or "chronic candidiasis syndrome." *Candida* hypersensitivity has been specifically suggested to be involved in MS. It is claimed that it may occur with MS because of MS-associated immune system abnormalities or the use of steroids, which suppress the immune system. In addition to MS, candidiasis hypersensitivity has been associated with fatigue, depression, anxiety, schizophrenia, rheumatoid arthritis, AIDS, breathing problems, and bladder infections. It is claimed that 30 percent of people in United States have candidiasis hypersensitivity. Demonstrating the presence of the organism is apparently not necessary to make the diagnosis. These ideas have been popularized Drs. William Crook and Orion Truss.

Treatment Method

Several treatment measures are often recommended for people with suspected candidiasis hypersensitivity. These include avoidance of moldy environments and dietary changes to eliminate foods that might contain yeast. Therapy may also involve the use of vitamin supplements and antifungal drugs such as nystatin, ketoconazole, or amphotericin.

Studies in MS and Other Conditions

There is no evidence that *Candida* plays an important role in MS or in conditions other than obvious *Candida* infections. No large clinical studies have shown drug or diet therapy for *Candida* to be beneficial for MS or MS-associated symptoms.

Side Effects

If *Candida* therapy is considered, it must first be discussed with a physician. The antifungal drugs used for this therapy are generally well tolerated. However, they occasionally produce liver inflammation, and in rare situations they have caused fatal liver injury.

Conclusion

Treatment for *Candida* should be approached cautiously. There is no strong evidence that *Candida* causes MS or that treatment for *Candida* improves the course of the disease or symptoms of MS. There is rare toxicity associated with the medications used for treatment.

Additional Reading

Journal Articles

Bennett JE. Searching for the yeast connection. *N Engl J Med* 1990; 323:1766–1767.
Blonz ER. Is there an epidemic of chronic candidiasis in our midst? *JAMA* 1986; 256:3138–3189.

Chelation Therapy

Chelation therapy is a procedure in which chemicals that bind metals are given for health reasons. This form of treatment has sometimes been claimed to be effective for MS. It is estimated that chelation therapy is used by tens of thousands of people in the United States for MS and other health problems.

Treatment Method

In chelation therapy, a substance called EDTA (ethylenediaminetetraacetic acid) is given by an intravenous infusion. EDTA binds strongly to (chelates) harmful metals, and the metal-EDTA complexes are then excreted in the urine. Vitamin and mineral supplements are also frequently given. A course of treatment may involve 20 to 50 infusions. This type of therapy is effective for known situations of heavy-metal toxicity, such as lead poisoning.

There are also chelation products that are taken orally. They are of no proven value, and the FDA has determined that they should not be sold.

Studies in MS and Other Conditions

Chelation therapy has been recommended by some for MS. Since 1955, some proponents have advocated its use for heart disease because it can presumably remove calcium from harmful "plaque" on blood vessels. Chelation therapy has also been recommended for people with strokes, Parkinson's disease, Alzheimer's disease, muscular dystrophy, heart disease, cancer, and arthritis.

The only clear indication for chelation therapy is heavy-metal poisoning. There are no well-designed studies to support the use of chelation therapy for MS, and studies in heart disease and peripheral vascular disease have shown no clear benefit for chelation therapy.

Side Effects

Chelation therapy has potential risks. Side effects include kidney injury, bone marrow damage, anemia, irregular heart rhythms, and inflammation at the sites used for intravenous lines. Rarely, fatalities may occur. Fourteen deaths were attributed to chelation therapy in one clinic.

Practical Information

Chelation therapy is expensive. A course of treatment may cost as much as $5,000.

Conclusion

There are no well-documented clinical or scientific studies that indicate that chelation therapy is an effective treatment for MS. Rarely, it may produce serious side effects, and it is very expensive.

Additional Readings

Books

Cassileth BR. *The Alternative Medicine Handbook*. New York: W.W. Norton, 1998, pp. 152–153, 176–178.

Dillard J, Ziporyn T. *Alternative Medicine for Dummies*. Foster City, CA: IDG Books, 1998, p. 42.

Spencer JW, Jacobs JJ. *Complementary/Alternative Medicine: An Evidence-Based Approach*. St. Louis: Mosby, 1999, pp. 92–94, 189, 403.

Chiropractic Medicine

Chiropractic medicine is one of the most popular forms of CAM in the United States. Chiropractors are the largest group of alternative medicine practitioners and the third largest group of healthcare professionals in the United States (after physicians and dentists). It is estimated that more than 160 million Americans visit chiropractors yearly.

Part of the popularity of this therapy in the United States may be due to the fact that chiropractic medicine, unlike many other forms of CAM, was founded in this country. It was developed by Daniel D. Palmer in Iowa in the 1890s. Some form of spinal manipulation, as used in chiropractic medicine, has also been practiced in other cultures, including ancient Egypt and ancient Greece.

Chiropractic medicine has been severely criticized by mainstream medical professionals. The American Medical Association (AMA) has long questioned the effectiveness and safety of chiropractic medicine. In the 1960s, the AMA passed a resolution banning physicians from association with chiropractors and established a board, The Committee on Quackery, to discourage the use of chiropractors. In 1990, the Supreme Court ruled that the AMA was guilty of a conspiracy to "contain and eliminate" the chiropractic profession.

Treatment Method

Chiropractors believe that mild bone abnormalities of the spine are the cause of many medical disorders. According to this theory, the function of the nerves that leave the spine is altered by "subluxations," misalignments of the bones of the spine. As a result, these bony abnormalities may produce nerve pressure, which may then affect many different muscles and organs of the body. This is sometimes compared to the decreased flow of water that is caused by standing on a garden hose and the increase, or normal flow, of water caused by taking one's foot off the hose. Chiropractors attempt to treat these bone abnormalities through a variety of spinal manipulation techniques, or "adjustments," which presumably normalize the bone positions. In addition to this theory of spinal manipulation, chiropractic medicine holds that the body is able to heal itself and discourages the use of drugs and surgery.

There are two groups of chiropractors, "straights" and "mixers." Straights use only spinal manipulation. Mixers, who represent the majority of chiropractors in the United States, use manipulation techniques and other measures, which may include ultrasound, massage, herb or vitamin supplements, and dietary recommendations.

Studies in MS and Other Conditions

There is no well-documented evidence that chiropractic therapy improves the course of MS. Studies of chiropractic medicine applied to MS are limited to isolated reports of individual responses to this therapy.

Musculoskeletal conditions that are seen in MS may respond favorably to chiropractic therapy. Most notably, multiple studies have evaluated the chiropractic treatment of low back pain, which may occur in people with MS. When it is of short duration (one month or less), low back pain improves with manipulation. Low back pain of longer duration may also respond to this treatment. Of note, besides chiropractors, physical therapists and osteopaths also perform spinal manipulation. In addition, low back pain may resolve with no therapy at all and may respond to therapy from primary care doctors, orthopedic physicians, neurologists, and physical therapists. The relative effectiveness and expense of these different approaches is debatable. In 1994, the Agency for Healthcare Policy and Research endorsed chiropractic therapy for low back pain that is recent and not long-standing.

The effects of chiropractic therapy on neck pain are less clear. Some studies have reported positive results, but this is less definitive than the studies of low back pain. Also, there is a rare chance of producing a stroke with manipulation for neck pain (see below).

Chiropractic therapy has been investigated in other conditions. Among neurologic disorders, there are small or single-case studies of beneficial responses in people with headaches and spinal cord injury. These studies are too small to be conclusive. Chiropractic therapy is sometimes recommended for many other conditions, including asthma, ear infections, and gastrointestinal disorders. There is no strong evidence supporting its use in these conditions.

Side Effects

Chiropractic therapy usually is well tolerated. Only 135 complications were reported between 1900 and 1980. Most complications are from neck manipulation. For people with serious diseases or symptoms, it is important to be evaluated and treated fully by a physician and not to substitute chiropractic medicine for conventional medicine. This is because chiropractors are not as well trained in diagnosis as physicians.

For people who pursue chiropractic therapy, one of the more common adverse effects is achy muscles, which may last one to two days after therapy. One significant possible complication is stroke associated with neck manipulation. This is very rare (1 in 40,000 to 1 in approximately 3,000,000), but it may also be very serious. Bone fractures and injuries to disks are also very rare. Injuries to nerves of the lower spine as a result of lower back manipulation ("cauda equina syndrome") are also extremely rare. Such injuries are estimated to occur in 1 of 100 million manipulations.

Chiropractic manipulation should be avoided by women who are pregnant and by people with spinal bone fractures or dislocations, spine trauma, severe disk herniations, cancer or infection of the bone, severe osteoporosis, severe arthritis, severe diabetes, and those undergoing treatment with blood-thinning medications.

Practical Information

Chiropractic treatment is often done on a weekly basis. Single sessions cost $25 to $40. Medicare, Medicaid, and some private health insurance plans may cover the cost of chiropractic therapy.

The amount of therapy needed depends on the individual and the type of problem. For low back pain, improvement typically starts within four weeks, and the entire therapy course generally lasts six to eight weeks.

Chiropractors are licensed in all states. More information about chiropractic medicine and practitioners may be obtained from:

- The American Chiropractic Association, 1701 Clarendon Boulevard, Arlington, Virginia 22209, 703-276-8800.
- International Chiropractors Association, 1110 North Glebe Road, Suite 100, Arlington, Virginia 22201, 703-528-5000.

Conclusion

There is no strong published evidence that chiropractic therapy is beneficial for MS attacks or altering the overall course of the disease. However, low back pain, which may occur with MS, responds positively to chiropractic manipulation. There is less supportive evidence that chiropractic therapy improves neck pain and headaches. Users of chiropractic therapy should be aware of the rare side effects, including stroke, and should rely on physicians, not on chiropractors, for diagnosis and treatment of potentially serious conditions.

Additional Readings

Books

Dillard J, Ziporyn T. *Alternative Medicine for Dummies*. Foster City, CA: IDG Books, 1998, pp. 139–152.

Spencer JW, Jacobs JJ. *Complementary/Alternative Medicine: An Evidence-Based Approach*. St. Louis: Mosby, 1999, pp. 140, 172, 299, 314–315, 376–377.

Journal Articles

Andersson Gunnar BJ, Lucente T, Davis AM, et al. A comparison of osteopathic spinal manipulation with standard care for patients with low back pain. *N Engl J Med* 1999; 341:1426–1431.

Kaptchuk TJ, Eisenberg DM. Chiropractic—origins, controversies, and contributions. *Arch Intern Med* 1998; 158:2215–2224.

LaBan MM, Taylor RS. Manipulation: an objective analysis of the literature. *Orthop Clin North Am* 1992; 23:451–459.

Shekelle PG. What role for chiropractic in health care? *N Engl J Med* 1998; 339:1074–1075.

Colon Therapy, Detoxification, and Enemas

Colon therapy has been practiced in some form for thousands of years. It was used in ancient Egypt and ancient Greece. The use of colon therapy in the United States began in the 1890s. At that time, it was often part of therapy that was provided at health spas. The popularity of colon therapy waned in the 1940s but has grown significantly since that time. It is estimated that tens of thousands of Americans are currently treated with colon therapy. Colon therapy is sometimes suggested for people with MS and also as a component of preventive health care.

Treatment Method

In colon therapy, the large intestine, or colon, is cleansed with liquid. Plastic tubes are placed in the rectum, and a solution, which may be water or water mixed with herbs or enzymes, is then passed through the tubing and into the colon. The solution is eventually passed through one of the tubes in the rectum. Whereas an ordinary enema generally uses about one quart of water, a session of colon therapy may use 20 or more gallons of water. Colon therapy sessions last approximately one hour.

Colon therapy is claimed to be beneficial because it involves "detoxification." It is believed that waste material on the walls of the intestine is toxic and that this material is absorbed into the blood stream and produces disease. This toxic material is removed though colonic irrigation, and beneficial effects are allegedly produced.

Studies in MS and Other Conditions

There are no studies to document that colon therapy is beneficial for MS.

Colon therapy does not appear to be effective for any other medical condition. Standard enemas are effective for constipation.

Side Effects

It is important to be aware of possible serious side effects from colon therapy. Intestinal infections may develop if sanitary procedures are not used. There are some well-known cases from the 1980s in which people died from severe intestinal infections following colon therapy. Besides infection, colon therapy may produce generalized weakness, worsen hemorrhoids, and cause perforations, or holes, in the intestine. Colon therapy may be more dangerous in people with known diseases of the intestine, such as Crohn's disease, colon cancer, ulcerative colitis, and diverticulitis.

Conclusion

Colon therapy should be discussed with a physician. There are no known beneficial effects for people with MS. This type of treatment also may produce serious side effects.

Additional Readings

Books

Cassileth BR. *The Alternative Medicine Handbook*. New York: W.W. Norton, 1998, pp. 179–182.
Hafner AW, Zwicky JF, Barrett S, et al. *Reader's Guide to Alternative Health Methods*. American Medical Association, 1993, pp. 293–295.

Cooling Therapy

Cooling therapy is a unique form of CAM for people with MS. Small decreases in body temperature may lead to relief of some MS-related symptoms. Cooling methods ranging from the simple to the complex have been developed. The use of cooling suits for MS was introduced in the United States in the early 1990s.

The effect of heat on MS symptoms has been known for years. Worsening of symptoms with small increases in body temperature occurs in 60 to 80 percent of people with MS. In fact, the "hot bath test" was one of the earliest tests for diagnosing MS. In this test, which is no longer used, people suspected of having MS were placed in a hot bath and assessed for any worsening of symptoms. Similarly, early in the course of MS, the only noticeable manifestation of the disease may be a symptom, such as weakness, numbness, or visual blurring, that occurs only in situations that increase body temperature, such as exercise, sunbathing, fever, or warm showers or baths.

While warming may produce worsening of symptoms, cooling may lead to improvement. This cooling effect has been observed with cold baths or exposure to cold air, both of which may produce short-term decreases in the severity of MS-associated symptoms. This beneficial response to cooling is the basis of cooling therapy.

Unlike some forms of CAM, cooling therapy has a scientific basis. Nerve cells with damage to the insulating part of the cell (the myelin), which is what occurs in MS, exhibit blocked conduction of signals with small increases in temperature. Thus, small decreases in temperature may facilitate transmission of nerve signals.

Treatment Method

Different techniques may be used to elicit cooling. Simple measures include taking cool showers or baths, sitting near an air conditioner, using an ice pack, and drinking cold liquids. More sophisticated approaches utilize a garment, such as a vest, that produces body cooling. Cooling garments may be "passive" or "active." Passive garments, which use ice packs or evaporation for cooling, are simpler and more portable than active garments. Coolants actively circulate through active garments, which may result in more effective cooling.

Studies in MS

Small research studies indicate that cooling produces improvement in MS symptoms. One of the older studies, reported in the late 1950s, showed that a temperature reduction of as little as one degree Fahrenheit led to noticeable benefits. A 1995 investigation of six people with MS showed that cooling primarily improved fatigue and leg strength (1).

In a 1999 Swedish study of 10 people with MS, cooling suits relieved multiple symptoms (2). Beneficial effects included improvement in walking, transferring, and urinating. Overall, there was an increased ability of people to care for themselves.

Preliminary results in other studies indicate cooling-associated improvement in fatigue, spasticity, visual changes, speech difficulties, sexual disorders, cognition, and coordination.

Although multiple cooling studies have produced positive results, these studies are too small and are not rigorous enough to draw definitive conclusions. Researchers at the National Aeronautics and Space Administration (NASA) have been conducting more rigorous studies to clarify the effects of cooling on MS. The cooling apparatus used in this research involves technology developed at NASA. In 1999, a large, ambitious study involving approximately 100 patients in six different MS clinics was undertaken to evaluate the effects of cooling on neurologic function. The results of this study are not yet available.

Side Effects

In general, the use of cooling garments is well tolerated. There may be a feeling of discomfort when cooling begins. Some people report that handling the garments is cumbersome.

It is important to keep in mind that there is individual variation in the amount of cooling and the extent of benefit. Some people exhibit little or no reduction in body temperature with cooling. In approximately 10 percent of people with MS, there may be a "paradoxical" response, and symptoms may actually worsen with cooling therapy.

Practical Information

Cooling garments are available from several sources and are manufactured by:

- Akemi, Inc., Houston, Texas, 800-209-2665
- Cool-Sport, Torrance, California, 310-618-1590
- MicroClimate System, Incorporated, Sanford, Michigan, 517-687-9090
- Steele, Incorporated, Kingston, Washington, 888-763-3538

Health insurance coverage for cooling garments may be available.

Conclusion

Limited research studies have found that cooling produces improvement in multiple MS-associated symptoms, including weakness, fatigue, spasticity, walking difficulties, urinary difficulties, speech disorders, visual difficulties, sexual problems, incoordination, and cognitive difficulties. Research is under way to examine cooling in more detail. This therapy is usually well tolerated. Cooling therapy may make the transition from unconventional to conventional medicine in the future.

Additional Readings

Journal Articles

Capell E, Gardella M, Leandri M, et al. Lowering body temperature with a cooling suit as symptomatic treatment for thermosensitive multiple sclerosis patients. *Ital J Neurol Sci* 1995; 16:533–539.

Flensner G, Lindencrona C. The cooling-suit: A study of ten multiple sclerosis patients' experience in daily life. *J Adv Nursing* 1999; 29:1444–1453.

Guthrie TC, Nelson DA. Influence of temperature changes on multiple sclerosis: Critical review of mechanisms and research potential. *J Neurol Sci* 1995; 129:1–8.

Ku Y-T, Montgomery LD, Webbon BW. Hemodynamic and thermal responses to head and neck cooling in men and women. *Am J Phys Med Rehab* 1996; 75:443–450.

Ku YT, Montgomery LD, Wenzel KC, et al. Physiologic and thermal responses of male and female patients with multiple sclerosis to head and neck cooling. *Am J Phys Med Rehab* 1999; 78:447–456.

Craniosacral Therapy

Craniosacral therapy, also known as cranial therapy, cranial osteopathy, and craniopathy, is a form of bone manipulation that is derived from chiropractic and osteopathic medicine. Dr. William G. Sutherland initially developed the technique in the United States in the early 1900s. A modified version was developed by Dr. John Upledger in the 1970s. Dr. Upledger currently provides instruction in this therapy to large numbers of healthcare providers through the Upledger Institute in Florida.

Treatment Method

Craniosacral therapy focuses on the bones of the skull, spine, and pelvis. Through massage, it presumably facilitates the smooth flow of the cerebral spinal fluid, a watery liquid that surrounds the brain and spinal cord. According to the theory, more freely flowing cerebral spinal fluid results in improved functioning of the central nervous system, immune system, and other bodily processes. Craniosacral therapists claim that they can detect rhythmic movements of the skull bones.

Studies in MS and Other Conditions

The basic ideas that underlie craniosacral therapy are not consistent with conventional understanding of skeletal anatomy or nervous system functioning. There is no evidence that impaired cerebral spinal fluid flow is a common cause of disease or that craniosacral massage significantly alters cerebral spinal fluid flow. Also, it is not clear that craniosacral therapy rhythm is a meaningful measurement or that it can be reliably detected.

In addition to the lack of scientific rationale for craniosacral therapy, there is a paucity of clinical research. Craniosacral therapy has not been specifically researched in MS. Beneficial effects are claimed for many disorders, including brain injury, spinal cord injury, pain, and seizures. However, these claims are usually based on the experiences of individuals (anecdotes) rather than formal clinical trials.

Craniosacral therapy should definitely be avoided in infants and children because the skull bones are not stable at a young age and manipulation could produce injury. Adverse effects of craniosacral therapy have been described in adults. Mild headaches were reported in one study of 55 people with mild head injury (1). In addition, three people, or approximately 5 percent, reported more serious side effects. These included dizziness and body stiffness (spasticity), both of which may be present in MS.

Practical Information

Craniosacral therapy sessions generally last 30 to 60 minutes. Therapy is usually performed by a chiropractor or an osteopath.

Conclusion

Most claims about craniosacral therapy are not supported by clinical studies. Side effects may occur in 5 percent of people treated. The theoretical basis for the therapy is not consistent with current understanding of the nervous system.

Additional Readings

Books

Cassileth BR. *The Alternative Medicine Handbook.* New York: W.W. Norton, 1998, pp. 222–225.
Spencer JW, Jacobs JJ. *Complementary/Alternative Medicine: An Evidence-Based Approach.* St. Louis: Mosby, 1999, pp. 172, 176–177.

Journal Articles

Greenman PE, McPartland JM. Cranial findings and iatrogenesis from craniosacral manipulation in patients with traumatic brain syndrome. *J Am Osteopath Assoc* 1995; 95:182–188, 191–192.
Rogers JS, Witt PL, Gross MT, et al. Simultaneous palpation for the cranialsacral rate at the head and feet: intrarater and interrater reliability and rate comparisons. *Phys Ther* 1998; 78:1175–1185.

Dental Amalgam Removal

The removal of dental amalgam has been proposed as a therapy for MS. This treatment is based on the idea that metal is slowly released from amalgam and causes or worsens MS.

Dental amalgam is composed of mercury as well as silver, copper, tin, and zinc. Amalgam has been used for more than 150 years to fill cavities and is used currently for 80 to 90 percent of tooth restorations.

Very small amounts of mercury are released from amalgam in teeth in the form of solid mercury and mercury vapor. It is claimed that the mercury released from amalgam damages the immune system and nervous system and thereby causes MS and other diseases. In addition, it has been proposed that disease is caused by harmful allergic reactions to the mercury or to the electrical currents generated by mercury. The presumed mercury toxicity is termed mercury hypersensitivity, mercury sensitivity, mercury toxicity, and micromercurialism. Electricity generated by mercury is called electrogalvinism or oral galvanism.

Treatment Method

A specific procedure is often followed when amalgam removal is considered. Questionnaires about symptoms may be administered. Electrical readings of restorations, skin patch allergy testing, mercury vapor tests, and hair analysis may be performed. Amalgam removal may be done by removing a few fillings at a time; this technique is claimed to release "locked mercury." Gold or plastic fillings are used after amalgam removal.

Studies in MS and Other Conditions

Dental amalgam has been implicated in MS on the basis of several weak observations. MS has been associated with both dental caries—the bacterial disease of teeth that produces cavities—and dental treatment. It has also been proposed that MS is caused by exposure to mercury or other heavy metals.

Dental amalgam has been implicated in many other diseases. These include diseases that may have an immunologic basis, such as arthritis, lupus, and chronic fatigue syndrome, as well as other neurologic diseases, such as headache, epilepsy, brain tumor, and Parkinson's disease. Amalgam has also been implicated in depression, cancer, and heart disease.

Contrary to what is sometimes claimed, there is research evidence that mercury from dental amalgam does *not* cause MS by a toxic effect. First, although mercury toxicity may produce symptoms that resemble those of MS, there is no evidence that mercury causes MS or that blood mercury levels are higher in people with MS than in the general population. Also, the amount of mercury released from amalgam is very low. Studies in the early 1980s indicated that relatively high levels of mercury are released, but subsequent studies demonstrated low levels of mercury release.

It is estimated that mercury from amalgam constitutes 10 percent or less of all the mercury consumed by an individual; other sources of mercury are food (especially fish), pollution, medications, paints, and disinfectants. For dental amalgam to produce mercury levels that are associated with even minimal toxic effects, it has been calculated that an individual would need approximately 500 amalgam surfaces or approximately 200 dental fillings.

Other studies also argue against dental amalgam playing a role in MS. People who believe their amalgam is involved in causing their symptoms do not have increased amalgam mercury release. Mercury levels in brain tissue from people with MS do not differ from those of the general population.

While there are anecdotal reports of benefit from amalgam removal, there are no well-designed studies demonstrating that dental amalgam removal improves the course of MS. Studies of large numbers of people with MS have not shown any association of dental treatment with MS attacks. MS occurred as a disease before the routine use of amalgam in dental practice and currently occurs in people who have no dental amalgam. Finally, dentists and dental staffs are exposed to relatively high doses of mercury and have blood mercury levels that are three to five times higher than the general population, yet MS is no more common in the dental profession than in the general population.

Professional guidelines do not recommend amalgam removal for MS. The medical advisory board of the National Multiple Sclerosis Society of the United States, the Public Health Service, and the National Institutes of Health do not support this treatment. In 1987, the American Dental Association determined that unnecessary amalgam removal is improper and unethical. In 1996, a Colorado dentist who actively performed amalgam removal on people with MS had his dental license revoked by the Colorado State Board of Medical Examiners.

There is no evidence that significant allergies to mercury cause disease. Allergy to mercury actually is very rare, and when it does occur, it produces swelling of the tissue around an amalgam-filled tooth and has not been associated with other diseases.

There are no large well-documented studies that have formally evaluated this treatment. In other words, no large group of people with MS has been studied to determine if removing amalgam produces a statistically better clinical course than not removing amalgam. Although the ideal clinical study has not been conducted, it is not clear that there is enough suggestive evidence to warrant the time, resources, and expense of such a study.

Side Effects

In general, dental amalgam removal is well tolerated. Rarely, it can damage nerves or tooth structure. For a short time, removal of amalgam may actually increase blood levels of mercury.

Conclusion

It is very difficult to determine with absolute certainty whether a compound such as dental amalgam is completely safe. The ideal clinical studies in MS have not been conducted. However, based on available evidence, there is no strong indication that dental amalgam removal has a beneficial effect on MS. Amalgam removal is usually well tolerated, but it may be very expensive.

Additional Readings

Journal Articles

Ekstrand J, Bjorkman L, Edlund C, et al. Toxicological aspects on the release and systemic uptake of mercury from dental amalgam. *Eur J Oral Sci* 1998; 106:678–686.

Fung YK, Meade AG, Rack EP, et al. Brain mercury in neurodegenerative disorders. *J Toxicol-Clin Toxicol* 1997; 35:49–54.

Mackert JR, Berglund A. Mercury exposure from dental amalgam fillings: Absorbed dose and the potential for adverse health effects. *Crit Rev Oral Biol Med* 1997; 8:410–436.

NIH Conference Assessment, Effects and side-effects of dental restorative materials. *Adv Dental Res* 1992; 6:1–144.

Sheridan P. Amalgam restorations and multiple sclerosis. *MS Management* 1997; 4:21–40.

Diets and Fatty Acid Supplements

$\mathcal{A}$ possible role of diet in MS was proposed more than 50 years ago. Since that time, this area has been a source of much controversy and confusion. Issues related to diet may be especially confusing for people with MS because some diet advocates exaggerate claims, and many healthcare professionals do not discuss the topic in much depth or with much enthusiasm.

A Well-Balanced Diet

It is essential to appreciate the basic components of a healthy diet before considering details about the possible influence of diet on MS. Regardless of an individual's specific diet, adequate amounts of a variety of foods should be consumed (Table 1). In general, eating a moderate amount of food from each food group should provide necessary nutrients.

Two Therapies Versus One Therapy

Diets and fatty acid supplements may affect MS by interacting with the immune system. Conventional medications for MS (Copaxone®, Avonex®, Betaseron®, Rebif®) also interact with the immune system. It is not known

TABLE 1. *Guidelines for a well-balanced diet*

Group	Daily Servings
Grains	6–11
Vegetables	3–5
Fruits	2–4
Meat	2–3
Dairy	2–3
Other (fats,oils, and sweets)	Sparingly

whether combining one of these conventional medications with a dietary approach would be beneficial. Because we have a limited understanding of the regulation of the immune system, it is conceivable, although unlikely, that a combination could be harmful. If a single approach is chosen, there is far more convincing evidence for one of the conventional medications than for a dietary approach.

Dietary Fat

A possible association of MS with dietary fat has been proposed. In the body, fats, which are stored in fatty tissue, are important for producing energy and providing the necessary chemical structure for the outer surfaces, or membranes, of all cells in the body. Fats are made up of *fatty acids,* long chains of carbon atoms attached to each other. Hydrogen and oxygen atoms are attached to these chains.

There are two types of fats. One is *saturated fat*, which is hard at room temperature and is what we generally think of as "fat." The fat that is on meat is one of the most important forms of this type of fat. Saturated fat is also present in butter and hard cheese. The fatty acids in saturated fats will not allow any more hydrogen atoms to attach to them. In other words, the fatty acids are already "saturated" with hydrogen.

Another type of fat is *unsaturated fat* or unsaturated fatty acids. Unsaturated fat is soft or liquid at room temperature and is frequently referred to as "oil." Examples of unsaturated fat include margarine and oils from vegetables, seeds, and fish.

The fatty acids in unsaturated fats exist in two forms. Monounsaturated fatty acids, which are present in olive oil, have one position at which hydrogen atoms may attach. Polyunsaturated fatty acids have two or more positions at which hydrogen atoms may attach. The body is not able to make polyunsaturated fatty acids. As a result, polyunsaturated fatty acids are essential in the diet and are referred to "essential fatty acids."

Polyunsaturated fatty acids have been the subject of most dietary studies in MS. There are two important forms of polyunsaturated fatty acids. One type is known as omega-six (or n-6), a term that relates to the chemical structure of these fatty acids. There are different forms of omega-six fatty acids, and these different forms may be converted into each other by a pathway of chemical reactions (Figure 1).

The first fatty acid in the omega-six pathway is *linoleic acid*. Linoleic acid is present in a variety of foods, especially the oils of seeds and nuts. It is converted to gamma-linolenic acid, also referred to as "GLA." GLA is not

Linoleic acid

↓

Gamma-linolenic acid (GLA)

↓

Dihomo-gamma-linolenic acid

↓

Arachidonic acid

↓

Prostaglandins and Leukotrienes

FIGURE 1.   *Biochemical pathway of omega-six fatty acids.*

nearly as common in food as linoleic acid. Relatively high levels of GLA are only present in unusual sources such as evening primrose oil. Further chemical reactions convert GLA to dihomo-gamma-linolenic acid and then to arachidonic acid. Finally, arachidonic acid is converted to prostaglandins and other chemicals that may be important for regulating the immune system and other body processes.

The other important polyunsaturated fatty acid is known as omega-three (or n-3) fatty acid. Fish and other seafood are the most well-known sources of this fatty acid. Once again, there is a pathway of different omega-three fatty acids (Figure 2). The first fatty acid in this pathway is alpha-linolenic acid, which is present in green leafy vegetables and flaxseed (or linseed) oil. Alpha-linolenic acid is then converted to eicosapentanoic acid (EPA) and docosahexanoic acid (DHA). Both of these fatty acids are present in fish and fish oils. DHA is converted to prostaglandins and leukotrienes, which are the same types of chemicals found at the end of the omega-six pathway.

MS and Polyunsaturated Fatty Acids

For years, MS has been associated with polyunsaturated fatty acids. In the early 1950s, studies were conducted in several countries to evaluate the possible impact of food intake on MS. Some of these studies suggested that

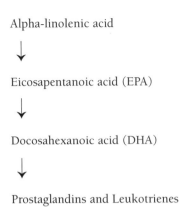

Alpha-linolenic acid

Eicosapentanoic acid (EPA)

Docosahexanoic acid (DHA)

Prostaglandins and Leukotrienes

FIGURE 2.   *Biochemical pathway of omega-three fatty acids.*

MS was more common in areas where the consumption of saturated fat, especially animal fat, was relatively high. Some research also associated MS with a high intake of dairy products. In contrast, in some studies, populations with a relatively high intake of polyunsaturated fatty acids, including vegetable oil and fish, appeared to have lower rates of MS.

As a result of the studies of polyunsaturated fatty acids in the diet of different populations, the actual levels of polyunsaturated fatty acids were determined in people with MS. Some, but not all, blood studies found decreased levels of polyunsaturated fatty acids, especially omega-six fatty acids such as linoleic acid. A few studies also reported decreased levels of omega-three fatty acids.

Many hypotheses have been proposed for the possibly decreased polyunsaturated fatty acid levels in MS. One hypothesis is that people with MS have some type of abnormality in the fatty acid chemical pathway. Another hypothesis is that people with MS do not eat adequate amounts of polyunsaturated fatty acids.

How could fatty acids have anything to do with MS? When the original studies were done with fatty acids, it was claimed that people with MS may have blood that is too thick and, as a result, flows slowly or "sludges." This idea is not consistent with our current scientific understanding of MS. It has also been proposed that, because polyunsaturated fatty acids are an important component of the lining of nerve cells (myelin), an abnormality of polyunsaturated fatty acids could produce abnormalities in the myelin, as is observed in MS. The current idea is that prostaglandins and other chemicals in the pathway of the omega-six and omega-three fatty acids (Figures 1 and 2) decrease the activity of the immune system. This immune-suppressing effect may be beneficial because the immune system is excessively active in MS.

Fats and Other Diseases

The effect of dietary fat on diseases other than MS has also been examined. Saturated fat, especially animal fat, increases cholesterol levels, and high cholesterol levels are associated with heart disease and stroke. In addition, some studies have associated high blood pressure and some forms of cancer with a high intake of saturated fats. Consequently, a diet that is relatively low in saturated fat and relatively high in polyunsaturated fat has general health benefits.

Specific Diets

The Swank Diet

Some of the original studies on MS and dietary fat were done by Dr. Roy Swank. Because of the apparent association of dietary fat with MS, he began treating people with MS with a specific diet in 1948. The diet involves a very low intake of saturated fat and a high intake of polyunsaturated fatty acids. Saturated fat is decreased to 15 grams per day. No red meat is allowed in the first year. Thereafter, 3 ounces of red meat per week are permitted. The diet does not allow high-fat dairy products or processed foods that contain saturated fats. High intake of polyunsaturated fatty acids, cod liver oil supplements, frequent meals with fish, and a multivitamin are also recommended.

In 1970, Dr. Swank reported the results of his diet in people with MS (1). On average, he observed patients over a 17-year period. People on the diet had less frequent and less severe attacks, less worsening of their overall neurologic condition, and a decreased death rate. The diet was reported to be most beneficial when it was started in people who were early in the disease course or who had mild disability. Some of the results were dramatic. For example, he described a 95 percent reduction in the frequency of MS attacks.

A follow-up report was made in 1990 (2). In this report, 144 patients were monitored over 34 years. Once again, the diet produced significant benefits and appeared to be especially effective when started in people who were mildly affected or were early in the disease course.

As noted, this diet is strict. Saturated fat intake is very low and polyunsaturated fat intake is high. Because of the decreased intake of meat, people who follow this diet should be certain that protein intake is adequate.

Most physicians and other healthcare professionals have a reserved approach to the Swank diet because the study was not carried out by guidelines that are now traditionally used in trials of new medical therapies. In particular, patients were not randomly given a specific therapy ("randomization"), the person who examined the patients was aware of their treatment (in other words was not "blinded"), and there was no placebo-treated group.

The Swank diet is a fairly extreme dietary approach without strong clinical studies to support its use. More details and specific recipes are provided in a book by Dr. Swank and Barbara Dugan, *The Multiple Sclerosis Diet Book.*

Other Low-Fat Diets

Other low-fat diets are more conservative than the Swank diet. It is not clear that the Swank diet is superior to these other low-fat diets; no clinical studies have compared the Swank diet with a less strict low-fat diet. General dietary guidelines that decrease saturated fats, increase fiber and polyunsaturated fatty acids, and maintain a well-balanced diet are outlined in Table 2. These guidelines are relatively easy to follow, are practical, and may produce beneficial effects.

The dietary recommendations in Table 2 have not been tested clinically. However, it could be beneficial for people with MS and may improve general health by decreasing the risk of heart disease, stroke, and possibly other conditions.

Other Dietary Considerations in MS

Constipation is a frequent complaint in people with MS. One way to improve constipation is to increase the amount of fiber in the diet. Good sources of fiber include whole grain breads and cereals as well as fruits and

---

TABLE 2. *General Diet Guidelines That May Be of Benefit for MS and General Health*

- Eat a variety of foods.
- Choose whole grain cereals and breads.
- Eat at least five daily servings of fruits and vegetables.
- Decrease total fat in diet to 30 percent or less of calories.
- Limit saturated fat intake.
- Eat fish two to three times per week.
- Choose a diet moderate in salt, sugar, and alcoholic beverages.
- Drink plenty of fluids and water.

vegetables. An increased intake of water and other fluids may also be beneficial for constipation; six to eight 8-oz. glasses of fluid daily are generally recommended. Some people with MS may have frequent urinary tract infections, and increased fluid intake may also be helpful for this problem. Finally, for some people with MS-associated fatigue, it may be beneficial to avoid large increases or decreases in the blood sugar level. This may be accomplished by eating small meals and snacks throughout the day.

Several other dietary factors should be kept in mind. Alcohol may, over the short-term, produce or worsen fatigue, bladder problems, walking difficulty, or clumsiness in the arms and legs. Grapefruit juice may increase the effects of many medications, including some that are commonly used for MS—diazepam (Valium®), clonazepam (Klonopin®), and carbamazepine (Tegretol®), sildenafil (Viagra®), and sertraline (Zoloft®).

Many diets have been recommended for MS with little or no supportive evidence. Avoiding foods that may cause allergies has been suggested. One example of this approach is a diet that does not contain gluten, a major component of wheat and wheat products. One clinical trial of a gluten-free diet in MS found no benefit. Studies of the blood and intestinal lining of people with MS do not indicate a sensitivity to gluten. There is no evidence to support the use of a pectin-free diet or a severely sugar-restricted diet.

If a specific diet is followed, it is important to always maintain a well-balanced intake of nutrients (Table 1). Some of the more extreme dietary approaches that involve a focus on one specific aspect of the diet may actually create problems by causing nutrient deficiencies.

Supplements of Polyunsaturated Fatty Acids

In addition to modifying the diet, the intake of polyunsaturated fatty acids may be increased by taking supplements. Some of these supplements have actually been studied in clinical trials of people with MS.

Omega-Six Polyunsaturated Fatty Acids
Linoleic Acid

Studies of Linoleic Acid.   Supplementation with linoleic acid, the first chemical in the omega-six fatty acid pathway (Figure 1), has been extensively studied. In EAE, an animal model of MS, supplements of linoleic acid are beneficial, whereas deficiencies of linoleic acid are harmful.

There are three studies of linoleic acid supplements in people with relapsing MS. Linoleic acid was given as some form of sunflower seed oil in these studies. All three studies meet the formal clinical research criteria of being randomized, blinded, and placebo-controlled.

The first study was reported in 1973 (3). Seventy-five people were studied over two years, and the daily dose of linoleic acid was 17.2 grams. Treatment produced decreased duration and severity of attacks. There was no effect on the frequency of attacks or the progression of the disease.

The second study was published in 1978 (4). Over a two-year period, 116 people were studied. As in the first study, the severity and duration of attacks were significantly improved, but there was no change in the frequency of attacks or the progression of disability.

The third study was also reported in 1978 (5). Seventy-six people with MS were monitored over two and one-half years. In contrast to the two other studies, no benefit was found in this investigation.

In summary, two studies produced limited positive results and one study found no benefit. To attempt to clarify the mixed results of these studies, a combined analysis was published in 1984 (6). The information on a total of 172 people from all three studies was pooled. It was noted that in the third study, which did not report any benefit, the people had more severe MS and had MS for a longer time than people in the other two studies. With the combined analysis, linoleic acid treatment slowed the progression of disability in people with little or no disability at the start of the treatment. Regardless of the duration or severity of the disease, linoleic acid treatment was associated with reduced length and severity of attacks. The statistical methods used in this combined analysis have been questioned. Overall, the effects of linoleic acid supplements on MS are suggestive but not definitive.

Sources of Linoleic Acid. Good sources of linoleic acid are the oils of seeds and nuts, such as safflower oil, sunflower oil, and sesame seed oil. Flaxseed (or linseed) oil contains linoleic acid as well as omega-three fatty acids (see section on omega-three fatty acids). Seeds and nuts themselves also contain linoleic acid.

A simple measure to increase linoleic acid intake is to increase the consumption of linoleic acid-containing foods, including oils. A more aggressive approach is to take oil supplements. The optimal dosage of linoleic acid is not known. In addition, the amount of omega-six fatty acids relative to the amount of omega-three fatty acids ("omega-six:omega-three ratio") is probably important, but the most desirable ratio of these fatty acids has not been established.

It is sometimes recommended that approximately four teaspoons of linoleic acid-containing oils be taken daily. The oil may be used in salad dressings or mixed in with vegetables, yogurt, or soft cheese. It should not be heated and should be stored under cool and dark conditions.

Risks of Linoleic Acid.   The most significant concern that has been raised about this type of supplementation is that it may increase the risk of cancer. This concern is based primarily on studies in animals. A 1998 review of all animal and human studies in this area concluded that it was unlikely that linoleic acid supplementation increased the risk of several types of cancer in humans.

There are other issues to be aware of with linoleic acid supplementation. The oily taste may be unpleasant, and diarrhea may occur in some people. Polyunsaturated fatty acids in general may produce vitamin E deficiency; low doses of vitamin E supplements may be indicated (see below). The possible adverse effects of long-term supplementation have not been formally studied and consequently are not known.

Gamma-Linolenic Acid (GLA)

Studies of GLA.   Evening primrose oil is a popular supplement that is sometimes recommended for MS because it contains GLA, or gamma-linolenic acid, which is one step beyond linoleic acid in the omega-six biochemical pathway (Figure 1).

There are some theoretical reasons why GLA may be better than linoleic acid, but there is scant clinical information in this area. A preparation of evening primrose oil (Naudicelle) was used in one of the linoleic acid trials in 1978. Eight capsules daily were not effective. In the same trial, linoleic acid alone was somewhat beneficial for relapsing MS. It should be noted that low doses of GLA (340 milligrams daily) were used in this trial, and it is possible that higher doses could have produced a benefit. However, this would have meant consuming up to 40 evening primrose oil capsules daily!

There are two other limited studies of evening primrose oil in relapsing MS. One of these studies also used a drug known as *colchicine*. Both studies produced some positive results. However, they involved a small number of people and did not include a placebo-treated group. Consequently, it is difficult to be confident about the results. A 1977 study of people with progressive MS found no benefit for evening primrose oil (7).

Scientific studies indicate that GLA suppresses immune system activity. In rats, evening primrose oil decreases the activity of *T cells*, a type of immune cell. GLA supplementation decreases the severity of disease in mice and rats with EAE, an animal model of MS.

Evening primrose oil has been claimed to be effective for many other conditions. Conflicting results have been obtained in studies of other immune diseases, such as rheumatoid arthritis, and in studies of premenstrual syndrome, heart disease, and a skin condition known as atopic dermatitis. There is suggestive evidence that evening primrose oil may be beneficial for diabetes-associated nerve injury (polyneuropathy).

In summary, the limited clinical information about GLA supplementation in MS does not strongly support its use. However, only low doses have been studied clinically, and scientific studies and clinical studies in other diseases suggest that it may be effective. In theory, GLA could provide the same benefits as linoleic acid, but high doses may be necessary and such high doses may not be practical on a regular basis because of its cost.

Sources of GLA. There are very few sources of GLA. Evening primrose oil is one of the most commonly recommended sources. It contains 8 to 10 percent GLA and approximately 70 percent linoleic acid. A single evening primrose oil capsule generally contains about 40 milligrams of GLA. Some capsules of evening primrose oil also contain vitamin E in low levels, such as 10 international units (IU) per capsule.

A 1992 Australian study evaluated the consistency of evening primrose oil preparations (8). Fourteen of 16 different preparations contained reasonable amounts (7–10%) of GLA. Because of the presence of other fatty acids in some of the capsules, it was proposed that borage seed oil (see below), another source of GLA, may have been added to these preparations.

If evening primrose oil is taken, approximately six capsules daily are often recommended. It should be kept in mind that GLA is present in low levels; six capsules daily will result in a daily dose of only approximately 240 milligrams. As a result, other omega-six fatty acids (see preceding) may need to be taken as well if one is attempting to significantly increase the total intake of omega-six fatty acids.

There are several other sources of GLA. Borage seed oil, which is sometimes recommended, is a rich source of GLA. It contains 20 to 26 percent GLA, more than twice the amount in evening primrose oil. However, borage seed oil may contain chemicals (pyrollizidine alkaloids) that are toxic to the liver. As a result, it is safest to avoid borage seed oil. There are some borage seed oil preparations that claim to be free of pyrollizidine alkaloids.

Like borage seed oil, black currant seed oil contains a higher concentration of GLA (14–19%) than evening primrose oil. However, this oil has not been well studied with regard to possible toxic chemicals or adverse effects. *Spirulina*, or blue-green algae, may contain high concentrations of GLA, but the amount of GLA in a given spirulina product is usually not specified and may be negligible (see "Herbs"). Finally, one of the more obscure sources of GLA is human breast milk.

In conclusion, evening primrose oil is generally preferred over other products for supplementation with GLA. Borage seed oil, black currant seed oil, and spirulina are of uncertain safety or contain variable and uncertain amounts of GLA.

Risks of GLA. In general, evening primrose oil is well tolerated. Long-term human studies indicate that a daily dose up to 2,800 milligrams of GLA is not generally associated with any serious side effects.

There are some concerns with the use of evening primrose oil and other sources of GLA. Because sources of GLA usually contain linoleic acid, the adverse effects and risks of linoleic acid are present. These include an unpleasant taste and soft stools or diarrhea. Additional concerns with evening primrose oil include expense as well as nausea and headache. Evening primrose oil and borage seed oil may provoke seizures in people taking antipsychotic medications. Evening primrose oil may affect blood clotting. Therefore, it probably should be avoided by people who take blood-thinning medications or high doses of aspirin, people who have blood-clotting disorders, and people who are undergoing surgery. The safety of black currant seed oil and spirulina are not known, and borage seed oil may contain liver toxins.

All supplements containing polyunsaturated fatty acids may produce vitamin E deficiency. Consequently, low doses of vitamin E supplements should be taken if vitamin E is not already present in the fatty acid supplement (see below).

Omega-Three Fatty Acids

Studies. There is one large study of omega-three fatty acid supplement use in MS (9). This two-year study, reported in 1989, involved 312 people and daily treatment with 10 grams of fish oil. The daily doses of specific fatty acids were 1.7 grams of EPA and 1.1 grams of DHA (Figure 2). People in this study were also instructed to increase omega-six fatty acid intake and to decrease animal fat intake. In the untreated group 52 percent worsened, while in the treated group 43 percent worsened. There was a trend toward a beneficial effect, but formal analysis showed that this effect was not quite statistically significant.

A small 1986 study evaluated the effect of cod-liver oil supplements, which contain omega-three fatty acids, on the MS attack rate in 10 people with MS (10). A beneficial effect of treatment was noted, but this study is limited by several factors, including the absence of a placebo-treated group and treatment that involved vitamin D, calcium, and magnesium in addition to cod-liver oil.

The study of omega-three fatty acids in MS is not an active research area at this time. However, other scientific and clinical aspects of omega-three fatty acids are under active investigation. Studies of immunologic function indicate that in laboratory animals and in humans omega-three fatty acid supplementation decreases the activity of several components of the immune system. In limited studies of EAE, an experimental animal model of MS, omega-three fatty acids have produced variable effects. Some studies actually indicate that omega-three fatty acids worsen the disease, but others indicate beneficial effects.

Studies of immune diseases other than MS have indicated a possible therapeutic effect with omega-three fatty acids. In people with lupus, as well as in animals with an experimental form of lupus, supplementation with omega-three fatty acids appears to be beneficial. Omega-three fatty acid supplements decrease joint stiffness and joint swelling in rheumatoid arthritis. Another form of immune disease occurs when organs are transplanted and subsequently "rejected." Omega-three fatty acid supplements appear to decrease the risk of rejection in both animals and humans.

Omega-three fatty acids may have other important health benefits. They have the potential to prevent and treat heart disease because they appear to decrease blood levels of triglycerides; inhibit "hardening of the arteries" (atherosclerosis); mildly decrease blood pressure; and decrease the risk of abnormal heart rhythms (arrhythmias), heart attacks, and death. However, fish oils may also mildly increase cholesterol levels. Fish oil supplements may be beneficial for people with diabetes because they have a favorable effect on blood levels of sugar and triglycerides. In spite of these suggestive studies of various health benefits, there is not a high level of interest in omega-three fatty acids in the United States. In contrast, there is considerable interest in these fatty acids in Europe and Japan.

Sources of Omega-Three Fatty Acids.   Fish is a common food source of omega-three fatty acids. Thus, a simple approach to increase omega-three fatty acid intake is to increase the consumption of fish, especially fatty fish such as salmon, mackerel, sardines, herring, tuna, or bluefish. Two to three servings of fish weekly are sometimes recommended.

Omega-three fatty acids may also be consumed as supplements. The optimal dose of omega-three fatty acids is not known. Also, the amount of omega-three fatty acids relative to that of omega-six fatty acids (omega-six to omega-three ratio) may be important, but currently there is not enough information to make specific recommendations.

Fish oil and cod liver oil supplements are available as liquid oil or as capsules. Concentrated EPA and DHA are also available. Total daily doses of 3 grams are believed to be safe (see below). One tablespoon of fish oil contains approximately 140 calories and 14 grams of fat.

A unique source of omega-three fatty acids is flaxseed (or linseed) oil, which contains both omega-three and omega-six fatty acids. The omega-three fatty acids are in the form of alpha-linolenic acid (Figure 2), as opposed to EPA and DHA, which are present in fish oil and cod-liver oil. (Interestingly, walnuts are also a source of alpha-linolenic acid.) The omega-six fatty acids in flaxseed oil are linoleic acid. Consuming flaxseed oil is a way to obtain both omega-three and omega-six fatty acids from a single source. One tablespoon of flaxseed oil daily is sometimes recommended.

Risks of Omega-Three Fatty Acids.   In 1997, the FDA determined that fish oil supplements were generally safe when the total daily intake of EPA and DHA was less than 3 grams. In one long-term study of 295 people, no serious adverse effects were observed with seven years of fish oil use.

Cod-liver oil has a fishy taste, and flaxseed oil has a bitter taste; these unpleasant tastes may be lessened by cooling the oils. Daily doses greater than 45 grams of flaxseed oil may have a laxative effect, and daily doses greater than 60 grams may theoretically increase blood levels of cyanide-containing compounds. Vitamin E deficiency may potentially develop when taking omega-three fatty acids; supplemental vitamin E should be taken (see below).

Most commercial fish oil products do not contain vitamin A. However, halibut, shark, and cod-liver oils contain relatively high levels of vitamin A. Excessive doses of these oils should be avoided because high levels of vitamin A may be toxic, especially during pregnancy (see "Vitamins, Minerals, and Other Nonherbal Supplements").

Finally, fish oils, specifically EPA, may inhibit blood clotting. These oils should be used with caution by people who are undergoing surgery, people who have blood-clotting disorders, and people who take blood-thinning medication or high doses of aspirin.

Vitamin E and Polyunsaturated Fatty Acids

Polyunsaturated fatty acids may decrease vitamin E levels. As a result, if high levels of polyunsaturated fatty acids are consumed in the diet or with supplements, vitamin E intake must be increased. However, *high doses* of vitamin E do not appear to be necessary. According to many recommendations, the ratio of vitamin E (in international units, or IU) to polyunsaturated fatty acids (in grams) should be 0.6 to 0.9. This means that, on a daily basis, 0.6 to 0.9 IU of vitamin E are needed for each gram of polyunsaturated fatty acids. Consequently, with an intake of 25 grams of polyunsaturated fatty acids, only 15 to 22 IU of vitamin E would be required. It is sometimes stated that hundreds of IU of supplemental vitamin E are needed if polyunsaturated fatty acid supplements are taken. This does not appear to be true. In fact, because it may be best to avoid high doses of vitamin E and other antioxidants in MS, as discussed elsewhere in the section on vitamins, lower doses of vitamin E may be adequate and may actually be more appropriate. Some evening primrose oil capsules contain vitamin E, in which case additional vitamin E may not be necessary.

Other Supplements Sometimes Recommended with Polyunsaturated Fatty Acids

In addition to vitamin E, several other supplements are sometimes recommended with polyunsaturated fatty acids. Vitamin B6 (pyridoxine) and zinc are recommended by some because the fatty acid chemical pathway uses vitamin B6 and zinc. In fact, the intake of these micronutrients from the diet is probably adequate, and, in the case of zinc, supplements pose a theoretical risk because they may stimulate the immune system (see p. 197). If these supplements are taken, the daily dose of vitamin B6 should not exceed 50 milligrams, and low doses of zinc should be taken (see "Vitamins, Minerals, and Other Nonherbal Supplements").

For antioxidant supplementation, vitamin C and beta-carotene are sometimes recommended in addition to vitamin E. As noted, only low doses of additional vitamin E appear to be needed, and there is no strong evidence that additional antioxidant vitamins are required. Because the benefits and risks of antioxidant vitamins in MS are not known, as discussed in the section on vitamins, it is not clear that vitamin C and beta-carotene supplements are beneficial. In fact, it is possible that, in higher doses, they may be immune-stimulating and therefore may negatively affect the course of MS. If vitamin C and beta-carotene supplements are used, they probably should be taken in moderation (see the section on vitamins).

In summary, low doses of supplemental vitamin E may be required when high levels of polyunsaturated fatty acids are consumed. It is not clear that there is a need for any other supplements, including vitamin B6, zinc, vitamin C, and beta-carotene.

Conclusion

Different Interpretations of Information

The area of diets and fatty acid supplementation in MS is controversial. This review of the positive and negative evidence shows that there are some suggestive studies, especially with omega-six fatty acids. However, these studies are not definitive.

With the information that is available, it is striking how many different interpretations and recommendations one can find. Some vendors of supplements and some books on CAM are overly enthusiastic about dietary changes, discuss only the positive results, and recommend diet changes and supplements for all people with MS.

On the other hand, more conservative conclusions and recommendations are made in the conventional medical literature. However, even within mainstream medicine, a spectrum of interpretations may be found:

- In an American text, *Merritt's Textbook of Neurology*, Drs. Saud Sadiq and James Miller write: "Diet therapy and vitamin supplements are frequently advocated, but no special supplementation or elimination diet has proved to be more beneficial than a well-balanced diet" (11).
- In a textbook on MS, Dr. Donald Paty, a Canadian neurologist who conducted the negative study of linoleic acid, states: "... perhaps [linoleic acid] should be reinvestigated in MS ... one cannot object to or condone such self-therapy ... one can understand the patient's desire to take a preparation that is not harmful if it might possibly have a beneficial effect" (12).
- A text by a Swiss physician, Dr. Jurg Kesslring, is more specific: "[The diet] can be enriched with cold-pressed oils which are rich in essential fatty acids ... vitamin E supplements are to be recommended ... capsules can provide, at best, a supplement to the essential fatty acids in the diet" (13).
- In a 1989 medical journal article, Dr. David Bates, who conducted several of the fatty acid trials, comments: "[T]here does appear to be a genuine, though mild, improvement with supplements of the diet by both omega-six and omega-three polyunsaturated fatty acids" (14).

Different Approaches

What is the correct approach in this area? Why are there so many different opinions? Much of the confusion and controversy in this area is due to a difference in perspective. Overall, there probably is no single correct approach. However, within a given perspective, there may well be a correct approach.

From a conservative, mainstream perspective, one would state that the results are not definitive and that no recommendations can be made until further studies are done. A more aggressive and unconventional approach is to state that the results are suggestive and that, because changing the diet and using supplements is probably not harmful, there may be some benefit to dietary changes and supplement use. These different approaches are outlined below.

■ *Conventional Approach.* Because the study results are not conclusive at this time, a conventional approach would involve no dietary changes or possibly modest alterations in the diet. No supplements would be recommended. This approach is often taken by physicians and other healthcare professionals and can be summarized as:

    ■ Diet—no modifications or modified as in Table 2

    ■ Supplements—none

■ *Unconventional Approach—Moderate.* Because of the suggestive results of the research studies, this approach involves some dietary changes and supplement use. This is an approach sometimes taken by people with MS who would like to make dietary changes and feel an urgency to act on study results that are suggestive but not definitive. This approach is:

    ■ Diet—modified as in Table 2

    ■ Supplements:

        – Omega-six—moderate amounts of sunflower seed (or other) oil and possibly evening primrose oil

        – Omega-three—moderate amounts of fish oil, cod-liver oil, or flaxseed oil

        – Vitamin E—as indicated

■ *Unconventional Approach—Aggressive.* This approach involves a significant change in diet as well as high-level supplementation. It generally is not recommended by healthcare professionals but is sometimes used by people who want to pursue all measures that decrease saturated fat intake and increase polyunsaturated fatty acid intake:

    ■ Diet—Swank diet or similar diet

    ■ Supplements:

        – As in Swank diet, also evening primrose oil

        – Vitamin E—as indicated

A Final Cautionary Word

There are several important considerations when considering any diet or fatty acid supplement use in MS. First, the prescription medications for MS

(Copaxone®, Betaseron®, Avonex®, and Rebif®) are more proven and effective therapies than diet or supplement use. *Changes in diet or supplement use should not be used in lieu of taking these conventional medications.*

Additionally, if diets or supplements are used in addition to the conventional medications, it is important to recognize that the effects of this "combination" therapy are not known. Presumably, two different approaches would be better than one, but the immune system and MS are not fully understood. It is conceivable, although unlikely, that a "combination" treatment such as this might be less beneficial than using conventional medicine alone.

Additional Readings

Books

Sarubin A. *The Health Professional's Guide to Popular Dietary Supplements.* The American Dietetic Association, 1999.

Swank RL, Dugan BB. *The Multiple Sclerosis Diet Book.* New York: Doubleday, 1987.

Journal Articles

Bates D, Cartlidge NEF, French JM, et al. A double-blind controlled trial of long chain n-3 polyunsaturated fatty acids in the treatment of multiple sclerosis. *J Neurol Neurosurg Psychiatry* 1989; 52:18–22.

Bates D, Fawcett PRW, Shaw DA, et al. Polyunsaturated fatty acids in treatment of acute remitting multiple sclerosis. *Br Med J*, 1978; 2:1390–1391.

Bates D, Fawcett PRW, Shaw DA, et al. Trial of polyunsaturated fatty acids in non-relapsing multiple sclerosis. *Br Med J*, 1977; 10:932–933.

Calder PC. Fat chance of immunomodulation. *Trends Immunol Today* 1998; 19:244–247.

Dworkin RH, Bates D, Millar JHD, et al. Linoleic acid and multiple sclerosis: A reanalysis of three double-blind trials. *Neurology* 1984; 34:1441–1445.

Horrobin DF. Multiple sclerosis: The rational basis for treatment with colchicine and evening primrose oil. *Med Hyp* 1979; 5:365–378.

Lauer K. Diet and multiple sclerosis. Neurology 1997; 49:S55–S61.

Manley P. Diet in multiple sclerosis. *Practitioner* 1994; 238.

Meyer-Reinecker HJ, Jenssen HL, Kohler H, et al. Effect of gamma-linolenate in multiple sclerosis. *Lancet* 1976; 10:966.

Miller JHD, Zilkha KJ, Langman MJS, et al. Double-blind trial of linoleate supplementation of the diet in multiple sclerosis. *Br Med J* 1973; 1:765–768.

Paty DW, Cousin HK, Read S, et al. Linoleic acid in multiple sclerosis: Failure to show any therapeutic benefit. *Acta Neurol Scand*, 1978; 58:53–58.

Swank RL, Dugan BB. Effect of low saturated fat diet in early and late cases of multiple sclerosis. *Lancet* 1990; 336:37–39.

Swank RL. Multiple sclerosis: Twenty years on low fat diet. *Arch Neurol* 1970; 23:460–474.

Enzyme Therapy

Enzymes are a type of protein used by the body to perform chemical reactions. Enzymes break down food in the digestive tract and carry out essential chemical functions in the rest of the body. It is claimed that treatment with enzymes is beneficial for many diseases, including MS.

Enzyme therapy has a long history. In one form of possible enzyme therapy, the Indians of Central America and South America traditionally use the leaves and fruit of papaya trees and the fruit of pineapples to treat inflammatory conditions. John Beard, a Scottish embryologist, first used enzyme therapy for cancer treatment in 1902. In the 1920s, Dr. Edward Howell claimed that consuming large amounts of enzymes was a way to help the body not deplete its own natural enzyme supply. In Germany in the 1960s and 1970s, enzyme treatment was recommended for MS, cancer, viral infections, and a variety of inflammatory conditions. Enzyme therapy was promoted by Drs. Max Wolf and Karl Ransberger.

There are two major types of enzyme therapy. In "digestive enzyme therapy," advocates claim that digestive enzyme supplements improve the breakdown of food, increase nutrient absorption, and decrease accumulation of toxins. Through these mechanisms, enzyme therapy is believed to effectively treat hundreds of diseases and maintain health. In the other type of enzyme therapy, "systemic enzyme therapy," it is believed that special enzyme preparations pass through the stomach undigested and then are absorbed into the blood stream from the intestines. Whether this process occurs and whether it offers any benefit is unproven. It is claimed that enzyme therapy has been used by many well-known public figures in the twentieth century, including Charlie Chaplin, Marlene Dietrich, J. Edgar Hoover, Aldous Huxley, members of the Kennedy family, Marilyn Monroe, and Pablo Picasso.

Enzyme therapy was under much scrutiny in the United States in the 1980s. In 1986, the FDA ordered one company, Enzymatic Therapy, Inc., to discontinue its publication, "Research Bulletins," because of false claims. Subsequently, the FDA continued to monitor informational seminars and material produced by the company. In 1992, the use of false claims by the company was prohibited by a court order.

Treatment Method

Most enzyme therapy involves taking supplements that contain enzymes obtained from animals or plants. Digestive enzymes from animal sources include proteases (chymotrypsin and trypsin), amylases, and lipases. Examples of plant-derived enzymes are bromelain from pineapples, papain from papaya, and ficin from figs. In Europe, intravenous infusions of enzymes or enemas of enzyme-containing solutions are also sometimes recommended.

There are rare situations in which enzyme therapy is used in conventional medicine. These conditions include pancreatitis, cystic fibrosis, and Gaucher's disease. An enzyme known as lactase is given for people who cannot tolerate dairy products (lactose-intolerance). People with excessive gas may find relief from Beano®, an enzyme (alpha-galactosidase) that improves the digestion of high-fiber foods, such as beans, peas, and whole grains.

Studies in MS

Specific enzyme treatment regimens, along with vitamin and mineral supplements, are sometimes recommended for people with MS. Surprisingly, some of these enzymes and other supplements are suggested because they *stimulate* the immune system. Despite the detailed and lengthy recommendations offered for MS, there is little evidence to support this therapy. No well-conducted studies of oral enzyme therapy have been published in English. A few clinical studies have been published in German, but they are difficult to evaluate because English translations are not readily available.

Intravenous enzyme therapy has been proposed for MS and other immune system diseases. It is claimed that intravenous enzymes may help break down harmful "immune complexes." A preliminary study in Austria reported some beneficial effects of this therapy in MS. Enzyme-containing enemas have also been recommended for MS, but no research evidence supports their use.

A clinical study is under way in Europe to further evaluate the effects of enzyme therapy on people with MS. This study is using a specific enzyme preparation known as *phlogenzym*, which contains a digestive enzyme (trypsin) and an enzyme from pineapples (bromelain). Animal studies indicate that phlogenzym decreases the severity of an experimental form of MS. The results of the human study of phlogenzym are expected to be available in 2001.

Side Effects

Oral enzyme therapy is generally well tolerated. There may be changes in the color, consistency, and odor of the stools when starting treatment. Excessive gas, nausea, diarrhea, and minor allergic reactions may also occur. Ulcers may be worsened by treatment with one class of enzymes, proteases. People with hypersensitivity to pork may not tolerate pork-derived pancreatic enzymes. The safety of long-term use of enzyme therapy has not been investigated. There is a theoretical possibility that long-term use could decrease the ability of the digestive system to secrete its own enzymes. Enzyme therapy should be avoided by women who are pregnant or breast-feeding; people who take blood-thinning medications; people who have blood-clotting disorders, severe kidney disease, protein allergies, and recent surgical procedures. With intravenous enzyme therapy, there are rare but serious adverse effects, including infections and severe allergic reactions.

Conclusion

In the medical literature published in English, there are no well-documented benefits of enzyme therapy for people with MS. Some clinical studies of enzyme therapy for MS have been published in German, but these reports are not readily available in English. Claims about this therapy may be exaggerated. The long-term safety of enzyme therapy has not been determined. Intravenous enzyme therapy may produce rare, but serious, side effects. A clinical study is under way in Europe to further evaluate the safety and effectiveness of enzyme therapy in people with MS.

Additional Readings

Books

Cassileth BR. *The Alternative Medicine Handbook.* New York: W.W. Norton & Company, Inc., 1998:183–185.
Sibley WA. *Therapeutic Claims in Multiple Sclerosis: A Guide to Treatments.* New York: Demos Vermande, 1996:59, 202.

Exercise

Exercise is not always classified as a form of CAM. Instead, it may be viewed as conventional medicine, or, entirely out of the realm of medicine, it may be considered a type of self-care or simply a component of one's lifestyle. Regardless of its formal classification, it is important to consider exercise because it is not always fully discussed during a conventional medical office visit, and it has significant health implications for people with MS.

Attitudes about exercise and MS have changed dramatically. In the past, regular exercise was not generally recommended for people with MS. However, based on more recent research demonstrating that exercise produces multiple beneficial effects, appropriate forms of regular exercise are now encouraged for people with MS.

Treatment Method

There are many possible exercise programs for people with MS. They may include stretching exercises, walking, running, swimming, and a range of other exercises that may be appropriate for all levels of physical functioning. In addition to these conventional methods, exercise may be obtained by unconventional approaches, such as yoga and t'ai chi, both of which are discussed in this book.

The specific type of exercise program that is best depends on the individual. Each person with MS has specific strengths and weaknesses, and these must be taken into account when developing an exercise program. An exercise program for a person with MS is usually developed by a physical therapist.

Studies in MS and Other Conditions

Exercise may produce a wide variety of health benefits. One well-known study conducted at the University of Utah was reported in 1996 (1). In 54

94

people with MS, 40 minutes of aerobic exercise was done three times weekly for 15 weeks. Exercise produced benefits for physical and mental symptoms, including:

- Weakness
- Impaired bowel and bladder function
- Fatigue
- Depression
- Anger

Similar findings have been reported in other studies. Also, specially designed exercise programs may improve walking steadiness, and stretching exercises may decrease muscle stiffness (spasticity).

Although exercise in general may be beneficial for bladder and bowel function, a specific type of exercise called Kegel exercises or pelvic floor muscle exercises may be especially helpful. With these exercises, the pelvic muscles that are used to voluntarily stop urination are flexed on a regular basis. These exercises are often recommended 60 to 80 times daily.

Although mixed results have been obtained, some studies show that Kegel exercises improve urinary function in both women and men by decreasing incontinence, urgency, and frequency. In some of these studies, the exercises have been combined with electrical stimulation or biofeedback (see "Biofeedback"). Further research is needed to evaluate their effectiveness.

Men with MS may experience erection difficulties. Research indicates that pelvic exercises may improve erectile dysfunction. However, this approach is not appropriate for men with MS because the beneficial effect occurs with erection difficulties that are due to blood flow abnormalities (venogenic erectile dysfunction), not for erection problems associated with nerve injury (neurogenic erectile dysfunction).

Studies in MS and other conditions demonstrate that exercise produces emotional benefits. In fact, more than 1,000 studies of variable quality have been conducted in the area of exercise and depression. One study that analyzed the results of 80 different clinical trials of exercise and depression found that the benefits of exercise occurred across a wide range of ages, in both sexes, and with all types of exercise. In general, longer courses of exercise (more than 17 weeks) are more effective than shorter courses. For treating depression, exercise appears to be as effective as psychotherapy and more effective than relaxation methods or pursuing enjoyable activities. Exercise in addition to psychotherapy is more effective than exercise alone.

Although anxiety has not been as extensively studied as depression, many studies have found that exercise reduces the level of anxiety. Many different types of exercise appear to be effective for depression, and longer exercise programs (more than 10–15 weeks) appear to be most effective. Surprisingly, individual exercise sessions that are only five minutes in length appear to decrease anxiety levels. Perhaps through these effects on anxiety, a regular exercise program may also improve insomnia.

Exercise has multiple actions on the immune system. The effect that these immune system changes might have on MS has not been studied. Moderate levels of exercise have been associated with immune system activation and decreased risk of viral infections, while strenuous exercise appears to produce mild immune suppression and an increased risk of viral infections. Because exercise has so many clear beneficial effects, the possible immune system changes associated with exercise should not factor strongly into decision making about exercise.

Other benefits are associated with exercise. Regular exercise may prevent *osteoporosis*, a decrease in bone density that may occur in MS. Low back pain, which may also occur in MS, may be reduced with an exercise program. Large studies have found that exercise decreases the death rate by 25 to 30 percent. This may be due to the protective effect that exercise has on heart disease and stroke. Exercise may also mildly decrease blood pressure, help prevent diabetes, decrease the risk of some forms of cancer, and improve symptoms of premenstrual syndrome.

Given the many emotional and physical benefits associated with regular exercise, it is possible that a lack of exercise, or "physical deconditioning," may actually contribute to MS-associated symptoms. Physical inactivity may worsen a wide variety of symptoms, while moderate levels of exercise may alleviate multiple symptoms.

Side Effects

The risks of exercise depend on the type of exercise. Increased body temperature with exercise may provoke neurologic symptoms in some people with MS. Musculoskeletal pain or injury may occur with overuse or trauma. The risk of exercise-induced injury is greater in those who are overweight, are older, or have had previous injuries. Finally, asthma may be provoked by exercise.

Practical Information

People with MS should develop an exercise program with the guidance of a physical therapist. This is especially important for those with significant physical disabilities or heart or lung conditions. Information on exercise is readily available from popular books and recreation centers. This information should not be used instead of consulting with a professional.

Conclusion

Exercise is a simple, safe, low-cost approach that may produce many health benefits. In addition to its positive effects on general health, exercise may have a variety of beneficial effects on MS-associated symptoms, including weakness, walking difficulties, muscle stiffness (spasticity), osteoporosis, low back pain, bladder difficulties, bowel problems, fatigue, insomnia, depression, anxiety, and anger.

Additional Readings

Books

Fugh-Berman A. *Alternative Medicine: What Works*. Baltimore: Williams & Wilkins, 1997: 94–100.

Journal Articles

Ernst E, Rand JI, Stevinson C. Complementary therapies for depression: An overview. *Arch Gen Psych* 1998; 55:1026–1032.

Petajan JH, Gappmaier E, White AT, et al. Impact of aerobic training on fitness and quality of life in multiple sclerosis. *Ann Neurol* 1996; 39:432–441.

Scully D, Kremer J, Meade MM, et al. Physical exercise and psychological well being: A critical review. *Br J Sports Med* 1998; 32:111–120.

Solari A, Filippini G, Gasco P, et al. Physical rehabilitation has a positive effect on disability in multiple sclerosis patients. *Neurology* 1999; 52:57–62.

Feldenkrais

Feldenkrais is a type of *bodywork* that focuses on efficient and comfortable body movements. It was developed by Moshé Feldenkrais, a Russian-born physicist. Feldenkrais is claimed to decrease stress, relieve pain, and improve balance and coordination.

Treatment Method

Very structured body movements are used in Feldenkrais. The position of the head is of particular importance. Feldenkrais usually is initially learned with lessons known as Awareness Through Movement (ATM), in which attention is focused on the motion of specific body parts during simple movements, such as walking or bending. In another type of Feldenkrais, Functional Integration (FI), more efficient movements are developed by a teacher who manipulates one's joints and muscles during movement. It is possible for people with significant disabilities to do Feldenkrais.

Studies in MS and Other Conditions

There are extremely limited studies that have formally evaluated Feldenkrais therapy. In a small study in MS conducted at the University of North Carolina 20 people with MS received Feldenkrais or a "sham" therapy for eight weeks (1). Some of the participants had significant walking difficulties and required the use of a cane or walker. Feldenkrais did not improve arm function, multiple MS symptoms, or overall level of function. It decreased stress and may have reduced anxiety.

Feldenkrais has undergone limited study in other conditions. Preliminary studies indicate that Feldenkrais may increase neck flexibility.

Side Effects

Feldenkrais is generally regarded as a safe therapy.

Practical Information

The cost of Feldenkrais depends on the type of therapy. ATM classes cost $5 to $10, while FI sessions are $45 to $80 per hour. Feldenkrais is usually not covered by insurance. However, insurance coverage may be available if Feldenkrais is provided by a physical therapist or occupational therapist.

Feldenkrais may be offered at local health clubs and recreation centers. More information and a list of certified practitioners may be obtained from The Feldenkrais Guild, 524 Ellsworth Street or Box 489, Albany, Oregon, 97321, 800-775-2118 or 541-926-0981.

Conclusion

In summary, Feldenkrais is a safe, low- to moderate-cost therapy that has undergone limited investigation. One small study in MS indicated that Feldenkrais decreased stress and possibly reduced anxiety. Further studies are needed to determine whether it has clear beneficial effects for stress and anxiety or for other symptoms, including pain, balance, and coordination.

Additional Readings

Books

Dillard J, Ziporyn T. *Alternative Medicine for Dummies.* Foster City, CA: IDG Books, 1998:171–172.

Journal Articles

Johnson SK, Frederick J, Kaufman M, et al. A controlled investigation of bodywork in multiple sclerosis. *J Alt Complem Med* 1999; 5:237–243.

$\mathcal{H}erbs$

$\mathcal{H}$erbal medicine has been used for tens of thousands of years. Neanderthals apparently used two herbs, yarrow and marsh mallow, for therapeutic purposes around 60,000 B.C. Within traditional Chinese medicine, herbal medicine was initially developed around 3000 B.C., and ultimately more than 10,000 different Chinese herbal formulas were compiled.

Herbal medicine was popular in the United States from 1820 to 1920. After 1920, herbal therapies were replaced by conventional medications. There has been a recent resurgence of interest in herbal medicine, and herbs are currently one of the most frequently used forms of CAM. The use of herbs by Americans nearly quadrupled between 1990 and 1997. In a return to earlier times, some major mainstream pharmaceutical companies are now developing and marketing herbal therapies.

Much of the popularity of herbs probably is related to the ease with which they can be used. There is no need to make an appointment with a practitioner to get started on herbal therapy. Rather, one can simply go the herb and vitamin aisle of the local grocery store or health food store.

Herbs have also become more popular since the passage in 1994 of the Dietary Supplements Health and Education Act (DSHEA), which loosened the regulations for dietary supplements such as herbs. In fact, the regulations are so relaxed that there are few standards for safety, effectiveness, or quality.

Herbs Contain Many Different Chemicals

An important distinction between drugs and herbs is that most drugs consist of a single chemical compound, whereas herbs consist of many different ones. Of all the chemicals in herbs, some may be beneficial, some may be harmful, and a large number have unknown effects on the human body. Fortunately, most of the chemicals are not toxic, and most are present in small enough quantities that significant harmful effects are unlikely.

Many chemicals with beneficial activity against disease have been identified in herbs. It is estimated that 25 percent of prescription drugs and 60 percent of over-the-counter drugs are derived from plants. Well-known examples of these drugs are digitalis, which is derived from the foxglove plant, and quinine, which is derived from South American Peruvian bark. Steroids, which are used to treat MS attacks, have a very specific chemical structure. Chemicals with steroid-like structures and biological effects have been identified in Asian ginseng (ginsenoside) and in licorice (glycyrrhizic acid).

Herbs may contain chemicals that have harmful effects. For example, the lily-of-the-valley plant contains potent heart toxins. Some herbs, such as chaparral and comfrey, have been associated with severe liver toxicity that has led to death or the need for liver transplantation. An example of a tragic case of liver injury was described in February 1999. A 28-year-old man with mild MS was treating his disease with zinc and two herbal medicines, scullcap and pau d'arco. He developed severe liver injury and died. The liver injury was believed to be due to a chemical contaminant in the scullcap.

Fortunately, most of the chemicals in herbs do not have toxic effects. For most herbs, the majority of the chemicals probably do not have any beneficial or harmful properties; if there are demonstrated beneficial effects of an herb, they probably are due to one or several of the many chemicals present. Thus, for many herbs, it is likely that one or a few chemicals could be producing a beneficial effect and that the remaining chemicals do not have any beneficial or harmful effects.

It is sometimes claimed that herbs cannot have harmful effects because the chemicals in them are present in such small quantities. It is also claimed that herbs have beneficial qualities. These two statements are not consistent with each other. *If a therapy is strong enough to produce beneficial effects, it usually is also strong enough to produce harmful effects.* As more research is conducted, it may indeed be found that, relative to prescription medications, herbs generally have fewer side effects but are also somewhat less effective.

Important Features of Herbs

Most herbs have not been studied as extensively as drugs. As a result, it is often not known exactly which chemicals in herbs are the active ingredients and the clinical benefits of herbs have not been as well studied as those of drugs. Similarly, the side effects of herbs and their interactions with drugs are not fully understood. In summary, even for the most well-studied herbs, the full range of effectiveness and the full range of side effects are not completely known.

Another important aspect of herbs is their variability. Because of the current lack of strict regulation in the United States, there is a great deal of variability in the quantity of the presumed active ingredient that is present in different herbal preparations. For example, one study of ginseng found 50 times as much of the active ingredient in some products as in others; this situation is similar to a physician telling a patient to take somewhere between one and 50 pills for a medical condition! Other reports have found no active ingredient in some ginseng preparations.

Finally, there are certain circumstances in which herbs should be avoided. People should avoid herbs if they have multiple medical problems or are taking multiple medications; women who are pregnant or breast-feeding and children also should avoid herbs. Some medications have a very specific range in which they are effective and in which they do not have side effects. These include anticonvulsant medications, blood-thinning medications, and some heart medications. Herbs should not be taken with these medications because we do not know all of the possible interactions that herbs could have with them. Some herbs could mildly alter the blood levels of these medications and thereby decrease their effectiveness or increase their side effects.

Herbal Therapy Guidelines

The most conservative approach to the use of herbs in MS is to state that they should be avoided entirely. The basis for this argument is that the effects of herbs have not been directly studied in MS and that it is therefore possible that an herb now thought to be safe could through future research be found to adversely affect the MS disease process.

For those interested in considering herb use, there are guidelines that can make decision making easier. These guidelines are outlined in Table 1. The final principle is very important—always discuss the use of herbs with your physician.

Choose Reliable Herb Suppliers

If using herbs, it is important to purchase them from companies that produce high-quality, consistent preparations. Many of the highest quality preparations are produced in Europe. Brands should be chosen that are standardized and contain specified amounts of active ingredients. The

TABLE 1.   *Herbal Therapy Guidelines*

- Herbs are often used as drugs.
- Herbs contain many different compounds, some of which may be toxic or interact with drugs.
- Herbs may contain compounds that have not yet been identified or characterized.
- The quality and composition of herbal preparations are variable.
- Herbs should generally be used for a short time for benign, self-limited conditions.
- Herbs should be avoided in women who are pregnant or breast-feeding.
- Herbs should be avoided by people who have multiple medical problems or are taking multiple medications.
- *Use caution* and discuss with physician before starting.

product should also list other specific information: common and scientific name of the herb, the manufacturer's name and address, batch and lot number, expiration date, dose recommendations, potential side effects, and quality control information. Higher quality herbal products in the United States have the symbols for the United States Pharmacopeia (USP) or the National Formulary (NF).

Consideration of Specific Herbs

There are many different herbal preparations. To provide practical information in this area, this section reviews some of the most popular herbs in the United States. Herbs with particular relevance to MS are also reviewed. These herbs are presented in alphabetical order. Following this section, both common and uncommon herbs are discussed in terms of their possible effects on MS and possible interactions with medications frequently used to manage MS.

Herbs Commonly Used in the General Population and Herbs That Are Relevant to MS

Coffee and Other Caffeine-Containing Herbs and Supplements

Coffee, perhaps not generally thought of as an herb, is in fact one of the most popular herbs in the world. Its effects on mental alertness and fatigue are well known to those who drink their regular morning cup of coffee. The effects of coffee are due to one of its chemical constituents, caffeine. In addition to coffee, other herbs and supplements contain caffeine.

Coffee is of interest for people with MS because of its possible effects on fatigue. There are no systematic approaches to using coffee or other caffeine-containing herbs in people with MS, and no recent studies have examined the effects of coffee or other caffeine-containing herbs on MS-associated fatigue. However, in the general population, there is strong evidence that coffee improves mental alertness, thereby potentially improving mental fatigue. In contrast, coffee does not appear to improve physical power or endurance and therefore probably does not have a beneficial effect on physical fatigue.

Another area of possible relevance to MS is immune system alteration by caffeine. Some studies indicate that caffeine may decrease the activity of lymphocytes, a type of immune system cell. In theory, this could be beneficial for MS, but studies in this area are too preliminary to allow any definite conclusions.

There are other herbal sources of caffeine. Tea contains a significant amount of caffeine. In the United States, black tea, derived from the leaves of *Camellia sinensis*, is the most popular form of tea. Green tea is prepared from the same plant, but the leaves are processed differently. Another well-known source of caffeine is chocolate and other food products derived from the cacao plant. Cola nut, also known as kola nut and bissy nut, contains caffeine. Guarana is a South American caffeine-containing herb that may be consumed as a tea or in tablet form. Another South American herb that contains caffeine, maté or yerba maté, is not especially popular in the United States but is popular in some South American countries. Finally, the most direct approach is to take caffeine itself, which is available in tablet form as a dietary supplement.

The amount of caffeine available from these products is variable. A convenient reference point to start with is a six-ounce cup of percolated coffee, which contains approximately 100 milligrams of caffeine. It is important to note that *less* caffeine is present in instant coffee and darker roast coffees, including latté, cappuccino, and other popular espresso-based coffees. In comparison to a typical cup of coffee, approximately one-half the amount of caffeine (30–60 milligrams) may be obtained from a cup of tea, cocoa, or maté; a 12-ounce bottle of a cola drink; or an 800-milligram tablet of guarana. Relatively low amounts of caffeine (5–10 mg) are typically contained in a chocolate bar. Caffeine tablets often contain 100 or 200 milligrams of caffeine and are roughly equivalent to one or two cups of coffee.

The FDA regards coffee and other caffeine-containing herbs as generally safe. One precaution to be aware of is the possible effect of caffeine on a developing fetus. Because of this concern, the FDA recommends that pregnant women avoid or limit caffeine consumption. Maté is an herb that has raised concern. The South American form, known as *Ilex paraguarien-*

sis, is generally believed to be safe. Past studies suggested that it may produce throat cancer, but this effect was later attributed to the high temperature of the tea, not its chemical composition. Notably, two North American forms of maté, *Ilex cassine* and *Ilex vomitoria*, are not classified as safe by the FDA.

There are some specific concerns about MS and caffeine-containing products. Caffeine use may worsen MS-associated bladder problems because it increases urination and may irritate the urinary tract. In addition, there are theoretical risks associated with the use of high doses of green tea. This form of tea contains relatively high levels of antioxidants, which may stimulate the immune system (see "Vitamins, Minerals, and Other Nonherbal Supplements"); this effect may be harmful for people with MS.

High doses of caffeine should be avoided because they may produce anxiety, insomnia, heart palpitations, upset stomach, and increased cholesterol levels. The long-term use of large doses of caffeine may lead to an addiction-type of situation in which higher and higher doses are required for the same effect and in which abrupt discontinuation causes mild withdrawal symptoms such as headache, irritability, and anxiety.

Caffeine-containing preparations also interact with other supplements and medications. Simultaneously taking moderate doses of two or three caffeine-containing supplements may lead to excessive levels of caffeine. Also, both the stimulant actions and the adverse effects of caffeine may be accentuated when it is consumed with ma huang (ephedra) or with grapefruit juice.

The usual maximum daily dose of caffeine is 250 to 300 milligrams. This is equivalent to two to three cups of coffee or four to five cups of tea. The timing and dose of caffeine that may be most beneficial for MS-related fatigue has not been studied.

Cranberry and Other Herbal Therapies for Urinary Tract Infections

Cranberry juice is of relevance because urinary tract infections (UTIs) are common with MS, and cranberry juice has a long history of use in their prevention and treatment. From the 1920s to the 1970s, it was believed that the acid from cranberry juice makes the urine acidic and that this increase in acidity fights UTIs. However, subsequent studies showed that the effect of cranberry juice was probably due to the presence of two types of compounds, fructose and a class of chemicals known as proanthocyanidins. These chemicals do not destroy bacteria. Instead, they appear to keep bacteria from attaching to the walls of the urinary tract. As a result, it is believed that bacteria present in the urinary tract are unable to cause an infection and are simply passed in the urine.

Limited clinical studies have evaluated the effectiveness of cranberry juice. One study conducted in 1994 found that consuming cranberry juice on a daily basis was associated with an approximately 50 percent reduction in bacteria in the urine. It is important to note that this effect was not observed until after two months of use. Several other studies of variable quality have also found beneficial effects of cranberry juice or cranberry tablets. A rigorous, well-designed study of cranberry use for the prevention or treatment of UTIs has not yet been done. Also, it is not known how the effectiveness of cranberry compares with that of prescription antibiotics, the more conventional method for preventing UTIs.

Because UTIs in people with MS may lead to serious complications, including worsening of neurologic difficulties, cranberry juice should not be used to treat infections. On the other hand, for people interested in an herbal approach, it may be reasonable to attempt to *prevent* infections with cranberry juice. The exact doses that should be used have not been established. Doses that are sometimes recommended for prevention are 3 (or possibly 5–20) fluid ounces of cranberry juice cocktail daily or 6 cranberry juice capsules daily (the number of capsules may vary with the manufacturer). A daily dose of 1.5 ounces of fresh or frozen cranberries is another option, but this usually is not practical because of the sour taste of the berries.

Another herb that is sometimes recommended for UTIs is bearberry, also known as uva ursi. There are some concerns about this herb. Specifically, its effectiveness has not been established, it appears to be less effective with acidic urine, and the possible toxicity of one of its chemical constituents (hydroquinone) has not been thoroughly studied.

Taking vitamin C supplements is a nonherbal approach that is sometimes recommended for preventing and treating UTIs. However, clinical studies do not support the use of vitamin C for preventing or treating these infections. In addition, there is a theoretical risk that high doses of vitamin C may stimulate the immune system and possibly worsen MS.

Echinacea

Echinacea is one of the most popular and most well-studied herbs. There is a long history of echinacea use for the treatment of medical conditions, especially infections. North American Indians used echinacea medicinally, and it was the primary herbal therapy for infections in the early 1900s. Echinacea poses a theoretical risk for people with MS, yet, surprisingly, it is sometimes recommended for MS and appears to be used by a relatively large number of people with the disease.

Echinacea is of interest to people with MS because it may prevent or reduce the severity of viral infections. Because viral infections may, in some instances, provoke an MS attack, their reduction has obvious potential benefit. Also, popular books on alternative medicine sometimes specifically recommend echinacea as a treatment for MS, possibly because of echinacea's effects on the immune system.

Many scientific and clinical studies have evaluated echinacea. Some, but not all, studies indicate that echinacea limits the duration and severity of infections, especially the common cold.

The important point for people with MS is that echinacea may act by stimulating two components of the immune system, *macrophages* and *T cells*. Macrophages and T cells are already excessively active in MS, and MS medications such as Copaxone®, Avonex®, Betaseron®, and Rebif® decrease their activity. Thus, consuming echinacea may conceivably worsen MS by further stimulating these immune cells and may impair the activity of MS medications. Another concern about echinacea is that it may produce liver injury when taken with methotrexate, a chemotherapy drug sometimes used to treat MS. *In summary, it is safest for people with MS to avoid echinacea.*

What about other measures to prevent or treat the common cold or other minor infections? Goldenseal and garlic (see subsequent sections) have not been shown to have definite effects on infections, and the scientific basis for their use is unclear. Also, vitamin C and zinc, which are discussed in detail elsewhere in this book, are sometimes used for infections. However, both of these compounds also have unclear effects on infections and may activate the immune system.

There are several measures that people with MS may take to prevent and treat viral infections such as the flu and common cold. First, the flu vaccine is readily available, appears to be safe for people with MS, and helps prevent the flu. Recently developed prescription medications also decrease the severity of the flu. Finally, viral infections may be prevented by simple measures such as avoiding contact with people with viral infections and frequent hand-washing.

Evening Primrose Oil

See "Diets and Fatty Acid Supplements."

Garlic

More than a thousand studies have evaluated the possible therapeutic effects of garlic over the past 20 years. Suggestive, but not conclusive, results have been obtained in studies of the effectiveness of garlic in treating high cholesterol levels, high blood pressure, and cancer. On the basis of limited scientific studies, garlic is sometimes recommended as a treatment for the common cold.

With regard to MS, some research has shown that garlic may stimulate two types of immune cells, macrophages and lymphocytes. No clinical studies have directly evaluated the effect of garlic on MS or other autoimmune diseases. However, garlic could potentially adversely affect the course of MS through its immune-stimulating activity.

There is controversy regarding the best form and dose of garlic. Some commercial preparations actually contain none of the presumed active chemical, *allicin*. Garlic may inhibit blood clotting and thus should be avoided in people with blood-clotting disorders, people undergoing surgery, and people taking blood-thinning medications or aspirin.

Ginkgo Biloba

Ginkgo biloba extract was the most frequently purchased herb in the United States in 1997. It has been evaluated in more than 160 human clinical studies and has the honor of being the most extensively studied herb. It is sometimes recommended as an herbal treatment for MS.

Much of the recent popularity of ginkgo biloba may be due to an investigation published in 1997 in the *Journal of the American Medical Association (JAMA)*. In this study, ginkgo biloba extract was found to be effective in treating cognitive difficulties in the elderly.

Several different biological effects have been associated with ginkgo biloba. Some of its chemical constituents act as antioxidants, while others inhibit the effects of platelet-activating factor (PAF), a compound in the body that plays a role in inflammation and blood clotting.

Because of the inflammatory effect of PAF, it and ginkgo biloba have been studied in MS. In animals with EAE, an experimental model of MS, PAF worsens the disease, whereas ginkgo biloba produces improvement. On the basis of these findings in animals, a small study, reported in 1992, examined the effects of ginkgo biloba on MS attacks and found that 8 of 10 people improved with ginkgo biloba treatment. Some herbal medicine and CAM books recommend ginkgo biloba for MS because of the results of this study. It is sometimes not mentioned that this encouraging 1992 study was, unfortunately, followed by a 1995 study that found that ginkgo biloba was ineffective for treating MS attacks. The 1995 study, which involved 104 people, was better designed and involved a larger number of patients than the 1992 study. Thus, *ginkgo biloba does not appear to be effective for the short-term treatment of MS attacks*.

There are some unanswered questions about ginkgo biloba use for MS. For example, could ginkgo biloba be helpful for decreasing MS disease activity when it is used on a long-term basis as opposed to short-term basis? Is ginkgo biloba effective for treating MS-associated cognitive difficulties? To date, research studies have not directly addressed these questions, and further research is needed to provide answers.

If ginkgo biloba is taken, it is important to keep in mind that it has a tendency to increase bleeding because of its effects on PAF. Spontaneous bleeding around the brain or in the eye has been described in a few patients taking this herb. It probably should be avoided by people who take blood-thinning medications (warfarin or Coumadin™) or aspirin, people who have bleeding disorders, and people who are undergoing surgery.

Clinical studies of ginkgo biloba generally use standardized leaf extracts. In these preparations, known in Germany as EGb 761 and LI 1370, there is a specific content of certain chemicals (24% flavone glycosides and 6% terpene lactones). Commercially available products with similar chemical constituents include Ginkai (Lichtwer Pharma), Ginkgo 5 (Pharmline), Ginkgold and Ginkgo (Nature's Way), and Quanterra Mental Sharpness (Warner-Lambert). Typical doses are 120 to 240 milligrams daily.

Ginseng

There are several different types of ginseng. Asian ginseng (*Panax ginseng*), is the most common and most extensively studied form. Asian ginseng was the third most frequently purchased herb in the United States in 1998. Another form of ginseng is Siberian ginseng or eleuthero (*Eleutherococcus senticosus*).

Both Asian ginseng and Siberian ginseng are derived from roots. They are "adaptogens," which means that they are believed to increase resistance to stress and increase energy levels. Although the effects of these herbs may be desired by many people with MS, it is not clear that consuming either of them is the best way to produce these effects.

Asian ginseng has been associated with many different biological actions. *Ginsenosides*, which may be the active constituents in Asian ginseng, have a chemical structure that is similar to that of steroids, which are used to treat MS attacks and *suppress* the immune system. Paradoxically, *activation* of the immune system has also been associated with Asian ginseng. Multiple studies have shown that the herb stimulates immune system cells, including T cells and macrophages. On the basis of these immune system effects, Asian ginseng has been investigated as a possible treatment for cancer and AIDS. Clinical studies of the effects of Asian ginseng on stress and fatigue have yielded mixed results. There is no clinical research that demonstrates that ginseng improves sexual interest or sexual performance.

Although Siberian ginseng is an entirely different herb from Asian ginseng, research on Siberian ginseng has produced results similar to that on Asian ginseng. Specifically, scientific research on the herb indicates that it may have immune-stimulating properties, and clinical studies do not definitely show beneficial effects on stress and fatigue.

There are possible side effects and drug interactions with Asian ginseng and Siberian ginseng. Paradoxically, both herbs may produce sedation and may conceivably worsen MS fatigue or accentuate the sedating effects of medications and alcohol. Asian ginseng may interact with steroids, which are sometimes used to treat MS attacks. Both Asian ginseng and Siberian ginseng may increase bleeding tendency and should be avoided by people who are undergoing surgery, people who have blood-clotting disorders, and people who take blood-thinning medications or aspirin.

It is reasonable for people with MS to avoid high doses and the regular use of Asian ginseng and Siberian ginseng because they may activate the immune system and they have not been shown to have definite clinical benefits.

Goldenseal

Goldenseal has been used medicinally for at least 200 years. This herb is taken alone or in combination with echinacea for a variety of infections, including the common cold. Unlike echinacea, which has been extensively investigated, there is little recent information about the biological effects or possible clinical benefits of goldenseal or its chemical constituents, berberine and hydrastine. Because of the limited information about goldenseal, it is difficult to make any definite conclusions about this herb. The clinical studies to date do not support its use for infections. Notably, goldenseal may produce sedation. Therefore, it may worsen MS fatigue or increase the sedating effects of alcohol and some prescription medications.

Grape Seed Extract

Grape seed extract use has recently grown in popularity. It is sold for its antioxidant activity; grape seed extract contains complex mixtures of chemicals known as oligomeric proanthocyanidins. These chemicals are similar to those in pycnogenol (see subsequent section) and act as antioxidants. Some studies indicate that the chemicals in grape seed extract are more potent antioxidants than vitamin C or vitamin E.

The clinical use of grape seed extract has not been extensively studied. For MS, it is important to keep in mind that, although antioxidants may have protective effects on the nervous system, they may also stimulate the immune system (see "Vitamins, Minerals, and Other Nonherbal Supplements"). Therefore, in theory, grape seed extract may worsen MS by activating the immune system.

If antioxidant supplements are taken by people with MS, it may be best to take low doses of inexpensive antioxidant vitamins, such as vitamin

A (beta-carotene), vitamin C, and vitamin E (see the section on vitamins). There is little or no reason to use a presumably potent and relatively expensive antioxidant such as grape seed extract.

Kava Kava

Kava kava is an herb that has been used in the Pacific islands for hundreds of years for its purported relaxant effects. It is one of the few herbs for which the active chemicals have been identified. These chemicals are known as "kavalactones" or "kavapyrones." Exactly how they produce their clinical effects is not known. Five German studies indicate that kava kava decreases anxiety; these studies have involved a total of more than 400 patients but are of variable quality.

Kava kava is sometimes recommended for insomnia. However, its effects on insomnia have not been well studied. Another herb, valerian, has been more extensively studied for insomnia than kava kava (see below).

Most drugs that decrease anxiety also produce sedation. Surprisingly, kava kava itself does not appear to have this effect. However, kava kava may increase the sedating effects of alcohol and several medications that are frequently used in MS, including lioresal (Baclofen®), tizanidine (Zanaflex®), and diazepam (Valium®). The effects of kava kava on MS fatigue are not known. Heavy use of kava kava over months may produce skin problems, red eyes, itching, and other difficulties.

Because anxiety may be due to multiple conditions, including medical problems, it should be evaluated and treated by a physician. Kava kava products should list the amount of kavalactones in each pill. Clinical studies on kava kava have used preparations with 30 to 55 percent kavalactones. Commercial products with a similar content of kavalactones include KavaTone (Enzymatic Therapy) and Kava (Nature's Way). The usual total daily dose is 60 to 200 milligrams of kavalactones, divided into two or three doses.

Padma 28

Padma 28, also known as Badmaev 28 and Gabyr-Nirynga, is a complex mixture of herbs that is sometimes recommended for MS. This herbal combination was developed in the late nineteenth century in the Buryat region of the Russian Empire by two physicians, Sul-Tim-Badma and Zham-Saram-Badma, also known as Dr. Alexander Badmaev and Dr. Peter Badmaev. The practices of these physicians were influenced by traditions of Ayurvedic and Tibetan medicine. Padma 28 is taken by mouth and contains more than 20 different herbs and calcium. It appears to have antioxidant effects and may mildly decrease immune system activity.

Padma 28 has been claimed to be effective for MS and other conditions, including heart disease, peripheral vascular disease, and asthma. In mice with EAE, an animal form of MS, consuming water that contains Padma 28 is associated with longer survival times and decreased death rates. A 1992 study in Poland evaluated Padma 28 treatment in 100 people with a progressive form of MS (1). Over the course of a year, one group of people received Padma 28 and the other group received no herbal treatment. In the treated group, 44 percent had some type of clinical improvement; none of the untreated people improved. This study is promising, but since specific details of its design are not available, the strength of the effect is not entirely clear.

The 1992 Polish study of 100 people reported no side effects. No other detailed toxicity information about Padma 28 is available.

Limited studies with Padma 28 suggest that it may be beneficial for MS. However, these studies are by no means conclusive, and there is limited information on the safety of this herbal preparation, especially for long-term use.

Psyllium, Bran, and Other Herbs for Constipation

Psyllium is an herb that is used for constipation. It is of potential importance to people with MS because constipation is a relatively frequent symptom of the disease.

Clinical studies have shown that psyllium effectively treats constipation. Unlike most other herbs, psyllium is approved by the FDA. It is referred to as a "bulk-producing laxative" because it increases in size, or bulk, when it comes in contact with water. Psyllium, probably the most popular bulk-producing laxative, is used daily in some form by approximately four million Americans.

Psyllium is a form of dietary fiber. Recent studies with psyllium and other sources of fiber have shown that a high fiber intake may improve several medical conditions, including high cholesterol levels, heart disease, and hypertension.

Psyllium is usually well tolerated. However, the FDA warns that it may produce choking, especially if the intake of fluids is not adequate or an individual has swallowing difficulties. Notably, some people with MS *do* have swallowing difficulties, and they should avoid using psyllium seed or husk.

Psyllium is available in over-the-counter preparations such as Metamucil®. It also may be taken in the form of the seed or husk. The FDA recommends that each dose of psyllium be taken with at least 8 ounces of water or other fluid. Oral medications should be taken one hour before or four hours after psyllium because psyllium may alter the absorption of these drugs.

There are other herbal therapies for constipation. One source of fiber is *bran*, the outer coat of grains, including wheat, oats, and rice. Bran may be consumed as a breakfast cereal, in tablet form, or as a crude material. Other fiber-rich foods include apples, citrus fruits, and beans. Other herbs that appear to be effective for constipation and are generally safe for short-term use (1–2 weeks) include buckthorn, cascara, castor oil, guar gum, olive oil, and senna. Long-term use of some of these herbs may lead to dependence on their use and decreased blood levels of potassium.

Pycnogenol

Pycnogenol has been used as a dietary supplement for approximately 15 years. It is made from the bark of the French maritime pine tree. Pycnogenol is a mixture of chemicals known as *oligomeric proanthocyanidins*, or OPCs. These chemicals, which are similar to those in grape seed extract and green tea leaves, appear to act as antioxidants.

Pycnogenol has been touted as a treatment for many diseases, including MS. At this time, however, no formal clinical studies have evaluated its effects on MS.

Pycnogenol may have several immune system effects, which may be the result of its antioxidant activity. As with other antioxidant supplements, it is not clear whether increased antioxidant activity is necessarily beneficial for MS. It is conceivable that antioxidants stimulate the immune system and thereby worsen MS. In this situation, antioxidant supplements with presumably higher antioxidant activity, such as pycnogenol, could actually be more harmful for MS than supplements with lower antioxidant activity. The safety of long-term pycnogenol use has not been documented in the general population. Pycnogenol and other specialized antioxidant preparations are generally more expensive than antioxidant vitamins.

There is no compelling reason for people with MS to use pycnogenol. There are no published clinical studies to support its use specifically in MS, and it carries the theoretical risk of stimulating the immune system. It is not known whether pycnogenol or any other type of antioxidant supplement should be taken for MS. If antioxidant supplements are taken by people with MS, it may be most logical (and most economical) to take low doses of one or more antioxidant vitamins, such as vitamin A (or beta-carotene), vitamin C, and vitamin E.

St. John's Wort

St. John's wort has been used for therapeutic purposes for more than 2,000 years. Its most common current use is as an antidepressant.

Although St. John's wort has been studied extensively, the chemicals that may produce its effects have not been clearly identified. A chemical known as hypericin may be responsible for its effects, but recent studies indicate that another chemical, hyperforin, is important. In addition to these uncertainties about its active constituents, it is not known how this herb alters brain function. Effects on neurochemicals, hormones, and even the immune system have been proposed. In the end, St. John's wort (and other herbs) may be found to exert multiple biological effects.

Many studies have investigated the antidepressant effects of St. John's wort. A combined analysis of 23 different studies that included a total of 1,757 patients indicated that St. John's wort had antidepressant effects similar to those of older antidepressant medications, the tricyclic antidepressants. However, the quality of some of these clinical studies has been criticized.

To clarify the possible role of St. John's wort as an antidepressant and to compare its effectiveness to that of the newer antidepressant medications (selective serotonin reuptake inhibitors, or SSRIs, such as Prozac), the NIH has funded a $3.4 million study of more than 300 patients. This study began in January 1998, and the results should be available in 2001 or 2002.

Because of the association of MS with depression, St. John's wort may be considered for use by people with this disease. No studies have directly evaluated its use in MS. Interestingly, one study showed that St. John's wort decreased the levels of interleukin-6 (IL-6), an immune system chemical that activates the immune system and may be involved in the flulike side effects of interferon beta-1a (Avonex® and Rebif®) and interferon beta-1b (Betaseron®).

Several factors should be kept in mind when considering treatment with St. John's wort. First, depression should be discussed with a physician because it is not a condition that people should diagnose and treat on their own. St. John's wort should not be used for severe depression (as opposed to mild or moderate depression). Although this herb is generally well tolerated, it may occasionally produce side effects, including upset stomach, sedation, dizziness, and confusion. Rarely, St. John's wort may produce sensitivity of the skin and nerves to sun exposure (photosensitivity), especially in fair-skinned people.

There are important potential drug interactions with St. John's wort. Because of its effects on the liver, St. John's wort may decrease the blood levels of a variety of prescription medications, including drugs commonly used to treat heart disease, depression, seizures, and cancer. Among these drugs of concern, several are used for MS-related symptoms: amitriptyline (Elavil®), carbamazepine (Tegretol®), imipramine (Tofranil®), nortriptyline (Pamelor®), phenytoin (Dilantin®), phenobarbital, and primidone (Mysoline®). St. John's wort may decrease blood levels of oral contraceptives and blood-thinning medication (warfarin or Coumadin™). In addition, because the biological effects of St. John's wort are not fully understood, the herb should not be taken in conjunction with antidepressant medications, including those referred to as "MAO inhibitors."

Tablets of St. John's wort are usually 300 milligrams and should contain 0.3% hypericin. A daily dose of 900 milligrams, or three tablets, is generally used. Companies that appear to produce high-quality St. John's wort products include Enzymatic Therapy, Indena, Lichtwer Pharma, Nature's Answer, Nature's Herbs, Nature's Way, and Rexall Sundown.

Spirulina

People have consumed spirulina, also known as blue-green algae, for hundreds of years. It was harvested from lakes near Mexico City by the Aztecs and from Lake Chad by natives of the Sahara Desert.

Spirulina is sometimes recommended for MS. It is also claimed to be effective for many other conditions, including fatigue, cancer, obesity, arthritis, viral infections, high cholesterol levels, and hair loss. Spirulina is also known as "super seaweed" and "superfood." It is rich in vitamins, minerals, and proteins and is available in tablets, capsules, powders, and processed foods such as snack bars. It produces a characteristic intense green color when added to drinks.

It is not entirely clear why spirulina is recommended for MS. Vitamin B12 supplements are sometimes suggested for people with MS, and spirulina contains a form of vitamin B12. However, vitamin B12 is probably not beneficial to most people with MS, as discussed in the section on vitamins, and apparently much of the vitamin B12 in spirulina is in a chemical form that cannot be utilized by the human body and could conceivably antagonize the effects of active forms of vitamin B12. Also, one particular species of spirulina contains gamma-linolenic acid (GLA), which could possibly be beneficial for MS (see the section on diet), but many other species of spirulina do not contain GLA, and it is not known exactly which species are present in a given spirulina product.

Spirulina may be associated with MS therapy because some studies have determined that it acts on the immune system. However, these immune system effects have been variable and of unclear significance; some studies indicate that spirulina stimulates the immune system and thus, theoretically, that it could actually be harmful for MS. Finally, spirulina may be recommended for MS because it is claimed to be effective for fatigue. No well-documented published studies support this claim.

In addition to the lack of evidence supporting its use specifically in MS, spirulina is relatively expensive and its safety is not known. Spirulina is at least 10 to 20 times more costly than other protein sources, such as beef and milk. There is insufficient information about the safety of long-term spirulina use. Although it has been consumed in some countries for hundreds of years with no apparent adverse effects, some batches of spirulina have been found to contain mercury, lead, arsenic, radioactive metals, bird feathers, flies, and microbes.

Stinging Nettle

The stinging nettle plant has been used traditionally in folk medicine. It is currently sometimes recommended for MS and many other medical conditions. Nettle is notable for having stinging hairs containing chemicals that produce skin irritation.

Nettle may have some therapeutic effects. For example, it may have anti-inflammmatory and pain-relieving actions. However, there are no clinical studies to justify the use of nettle for MS. In addition, scientific studies indicate that nettle may activate immune system cells (T cells), which poses a theoretical risk for people with MS.

The safety of nettle has not been extensively studied. In the United States, it is classified as an herb of "undefined safety." Nettle may produce sedation and thus has the potential to worsen MS fatigue and increase the effects of sedating medications and alcohol. Because of its vitamin K content, nettle may interfere with the effects of blood-thinning medications such as warfarin or Coumadin™.

Valerian

Valerian has been used as a sedating and calming herb for over 1,000 years. It is sometimes referred to as "the Valium of the nineteenth century." Valerian has a characteristic odor, which is similar to that of dirty socks. Different valerian products have sometimes actually been evaluated on the basis of their "stink rating."

Valerian may produce its effects by an action similar to that of Valium® and related prescription drugs (benzodiazepines). However, the active chemicals and their exact biological activities have not been determined. Ten clinical studies over the past 20 years have suggested that valerian is effective for insomnia.

Valerian is sometimes suggested as a treatment for anxiety. However, most of the clinical studies of valerian have been for insomnia. For anxiety, there are more extensive studies of kava kava (see preceding section) than valerian.

Sleep disorders are common in MS and may contribute to MS-associated fatigue. Sleeping difficulties may be associated with stress and anxiety. Because of the complexities of diagnosing and treating sleep disorders, this condition should be discussed with a physician.

Although valerian is usually well tolerated, the safety of long-term use has not been established. Valerian may produce excessive sedation or worsen MS fatigue, especially if it is used in combination with other sedating medications (such as Baclofen®, Zanaflex®, Valium®) or with alcohol.

Variable doses are given for valerian products. In clinical studies, the range of doses has been 400 to 1,200 milligrams, taken one hour before bedtime. The therapeutic effects of valerian may require daily use for two to four weeks (as opposed to sporadic use on an "as needed" basis).

Yohimbe and Yohimbine

Yohimbe refers to the bark obtained from a West African tree, which traditionally has been used for sexual disorders and as an aphrodisiac. Yohimbine is one the major chemicals present in yohimbe.

Limited studies have evaluated the effectiveness and safety of yohimbe for sexual disorders. Some studies indicate that yohimbe may be beneficial for erectile dysfunction. However, it has many significant side effects, including severe anxiety, other psychiatric difficulties, high blood pressure, and worsening of liver or kidney disease. The FDA has determined that yohimbe is not safe or effective and that it should not be available for over-the-counter use. Yohimbine, the active ingredient in yohimbe, is available by prescription in the United States.

People with MS may experience sexual disorders, including difficulties with erections and decreased libido. These sexual problems should be evaluated and treated by a physician or other healthcare professional. Yohimbine should only be used with physician supervision. For sexual disorders, conventional medical treatment, especially sildenafil (Viagra®) in the case of erection problems, is safer and more effective than yohimbe or yohimbine.

Herbs That May Affect MS, Interact with Medications Used in MS, or Have Serious Side Effects

Many different herbs are available in the United States, especially in stores that specialize in herbal products. Their beneficial effects are sometimes described extensively, while the possible harmful effects on a specific disease such as MS are not mentioned. In this section, we consider herbs that may stimulate the immune system, worsen MS-associated symptoms, and interact with medications commonly used for MS. Potentially dangerous herbs are also discussed.

Immune-Stimulating Herbs

In scientific studies, many herbs have been shown to potentially activate the immune system (Table 2). Apparently some of these herbs stimulate immune system function through a type of sugar molecule known as a "polysaccharide."

The immune system has two components, the *cellular* immune system and the *humoral* immune system. The immune-stimulating effects of herbs may be on one or both of these components. While much MS research focuses on abnormalities in the cellular system, both the cellular and humoral systems appear to be involved in the disease process.

It is important to note that the effects of these herbs on MS itself have never been specifically studied. The immune-stimulating effects have been shown in scientific studies, such as test tube experiments or animal studies. However, it is not clear how these effects in scientific studies translate into human clinical effects. In other words, it is not known whether an herb that produces an immune effect in a scientific study will necessarily cause any significant effect in a person with an immune system–related disease such as MS. It is also important to note that there are only a few scientific studies for some of the herb effects on the immune system. As a result, *much more research needs to be done* to more fully understand how these herbs affect immune function and how they might possibly affect MS disease activity.

Many commonly used herbs may stimulate the immune system (Table 2). Echinacea is the most well known of these herbs. Some of the other herbs in this category are among the most popular herbs in the United States, including alfalfa, Asian ginseng, astragalus, cat's claw, garlic, saw palmetto, and Siberian ginseng. Other immune-stimulating herbs may be found in this book in the sections on Asian herbal medicine and Ayurvedic medicine.

TABLE 2. *Herbs That May Stimulate the Immune System*

Alfalfa	Celandine	Licorice
Arnica	Drosera	Mistletoe
Astragalus	Echinacea	Reishi mushroom
Boneset	Garlic	Saw palmetto
Calendula	Ginseng, Asian	Shiitake mushroom
Cat's claw	Ginseng, Siberian	Stinging nettle

For people with MS, the use of an uncommon herb, woody night-shade stem, is specifically discouraged in *The German Commission E Monographs*, an authoritative text on herbal medicine (2). It is not clear if this recommendation is based on any possible immune effects of woody nightshade stem.

An error is made in some books about MS and herbal therapy. In these books, MS is described as an immune disorder. It is then assumed that MS is caused by *too little* immune system activity and that immune-stimulating herbs are beneficial. Consequently, some of the herbs in Table 2 are often *recommended* for MS. In fact, MS is an immune disorder, but it is caused by *excessive* immune system activity. Thus, on a theoretical basis, immune-stimulating herbs may worsen the disease.

It is impossible to develop strict guidelines about the use of these herbs because their exact effects on MS are not known. It may be best for people with MS to simply avoid these herbs. If they are used, they probably should not be used in high doses or on a long-term basis.

Sedating Herbs

Many herbs may produce sedation (Table 3). Some of the more common herbs on this list are Asian ginseng, chamomile, goldenseal, kava kava, St. John's wort, Siberian ginseng, and valerian.

The sedating effects of these herbs may occur when they are taken alone or in combination with sedating medication or alcohol. This is important for MS because fatigue is common in this disease. In addition, medications with possible sedating effects are used commonly in MS, including Baclofen®, Zanaflex®, Valium®, and Klonopin®.

TABLE 3. *Herbs with Possible Sedating Effects*

Balm	Ginseng, Asian	St. John's wort
Barberry	Ginseng, Siberian	Sage
Black cohosh	Goldenseal	Sassafras
Calamus	Gotu kola (hydrocotyle)	Scullcap
Calendula	Henbane	Shepherd's purse
California poppy	Hops	Stinging nettle
Capsicum (cayenne)	Jamaica dogwood	Valerian
Catnip	Kava kava	Wild carrot
Celery	Lavender	Wild lettuce
Chamomile	Lemon balm	Withania (ashwagandha)
Couchgrass	Motherwort	Yerba mansa
Elecampine	Passionflower	

Herbs to Avoid with Urinary Tract Infections

Some herbs may irritate the urinary tract (Table 4). The most common herb on this list is coffee. The herbs in this category may worsen the effects of urinary tract infections, which occur frequently in some women with MS. In addition, frequent use or high doses of these herbs may irritate the urinary tract even when an infection does not exist (3).

Herbs That May Interact with Steroids

Steroids are sometimes used to treat MS attacks. Some herbs (Table 5) should probably be avoided with steroid use because they may worsen steroid side effects (increase blood sugar or decrease blood potassium) or increase the potency of the steroids. The more common herbs on this list are Asian ginseng, ephedra (ma huang), licorice, and senna.

Herbs That May Interact with Antidepressant Medications

A class of older antidepressant medications is known as *tricyclic antide-pressants*. These drugs, which include amitriptyline (Elavil®) and nor-triptyline (Pamelor®), are used in MS for depression or pain. With these antidepressants, one should avoid St. John's wort, belladonna, henbane, mistletoe, and scopolia. St. John's wort also should be avoided when tak-ing the newer antidepressants (known as SSRIs), such as Prozac®, Zoloft®, and Paxil®.

Herbs That May Interact with Amantadine

Amantadine is used frequently in MS to treat fatigue. Confusion or seda-tion may occur if amantadine is taken along with belladonna, henbane, pheasant's eye, or scopolia.

TABLE 4.   *Herbs That May Irritate the Urinary Tract*

Asiatic dogwood	Eucalyptus	Pine needles
Asparagus	Fragrant sumach	Rue
Buchu	Guarana	Sandalwood
Celery	Horseradish	Sassafras
Cinnamon	Juniper berries	Tea
Coffee	Lovage	Thyme
Cola nut	Maté	Watercress
Copaiba oleoresin	Myrrh gum	Yellow cedar
Cubeb	Parsley	Yerba mansa
Dill seed	Pennyroyal	

TABLE 5. *Herbs That May Interact with Steroids*

Aloe	Figwort
Bayberry	Ginseng, Asian
Buckthorn	Gotu kola (hydrocotyle)
Cascara sagrada	Licorice
Devil's claw	Lily-of-the-valley
Elecampine	Pheasant's eye
Ephedra (ma huang)	Senna
Fenugreek	Squill

Herbs That May Interact with Methotrexate

Methotrexate is a chemotherapy drug sometimes used to treat MS. It may produce adverse effects if taken with aspirin-like chemicals known as *salicylates*. Herbs that contain salicylates should be avoided when taking methotrexate. These include black cohosh, meadowsweet, poplar, sweet birch, willow, and wintergreen. Another herb, echinacea, may produce liver toxicity when taken in combination with methotrexate.

Potentially Dangerous Herbs or Herbs with Unstudied Toxicity

Some herbs have been associated with significant toxic effects or have not been subjected to toxicity evaluations (Table 6). These herbs should be avoided. In spite of reports of toxicity, it is possible to purchase many of these herbs in the United States.

Potentially dangerous herbs that are sometimes specifically recommended for MS include borage seed oil, chaparral, comfrey, lobelia, and yohimbe. Borage seed oil, chaparral, and comfrey may contain chemicals that are toxic to the liver. Lobelia may potentially cause a rapid heart rate, low blood pressure, seizures, coma, or death. As described previously, yohimbe may produce psychiatric problems, high blood pressure, and worsening of liver or kidney disease.

TABLE 6. *Herbs with Potential Toxicity or Uninvestigated Toxicity*

Angelica	Dong-quai	Lobelia	Sage
Blue cohosh	Ephedra (ma huang)	Mistletoe	Sassafras
Borage	Foxglove	Muira puama	Scullcap
Calamus	Garcinia	Pangamic acid	Suma
Chaparral	Germander	Pau d'arco	Tansy
Coltsfoot	Kombucha	Pennyroyal	Wormwood
Comfrey	Life root	Rue	Yohimbe

Another herb in this category, ephedra (ma huang), is not generally discussed in the context of MS, but it is used fairly frequently. Ephedra may cause dizziness, irritability, headache, upset stomach, and heart palpitations. Rarely, its use has been associated with severely increased blood pressure, abnormal heart rhythms, heart failure, and death.

Conclusion

Herbs should be used with caution by people with MS. There are many herbs with no well-documented benefits that may potentially worsen MS or interact with MS medications. Some herbs may be of benefit for specific MS-related symptoms. These include St. John's wort for depression, kava kava for anxiety, valerian for insomnia, cranberry for the prevention of urinary tract infections, and psyllium for constipation.

Although some information is available about herbs and MS, much more remains to be learned, even for the well-studied herbs such as echinacea and St. John's wort. In a sense, the message for herbs and MS is similar to that for unconventional medicine and MS as a whole: some of the therapies may be beneficial, some may be harmful, and nearly all are not fully understood.

Additional Readings

Books

Blumenthal M (ed.). *The Complete German Commission E Monographs: Therapeutic Guide to Herbal Medicines.* Austin: American Botanical Council, 1998.

Brinker F. *Herb Contraindications and Drug Interactions.* Oregon: Eclectic Medical Publishers, 1998.

Foster SE, Tyler VE. *Tyler's Honest Herbal.* Haworth Herbal Press, 1999.

Jellin JM, Batz F, Hitchens K, et al. *Natural Medicines Comprehensive Database.* Therapeutic Research Faculty, 1999.

Newall CA, Anderson LA, Phillipson JD. *Herbal Medicines: A Guide for Health-Care Professionals.* London: The Pharmaceutical Press, 1996.

Robbers JE, Tyler VE. *Tyler's Herbs of Choice.* Haworth Herbal Press, 1999.

Sarubin A. *The Health Professional's Guide to Popular Dietary Supplements.* The American Dietetic Association, 2000.

Schulz V, Hansel R, Tyler VE. *Rational Phytotherpy: A Physicians' Guide to Herbal Medicine.* Berlin: Springer-Verlag Berlin Heidelberg, 1998.

Hippotherapy and Therapeutic Horseback Riding

*H*ippotherapy is an unusual term that refers to the use of horseback riding for therapeutic effects. The word is derived from the Greek word *hippos*, which means horse. Therapeutic horseback riding, a technique related to hippotherapy, aims to both produce therapeutic effects and teach riding skills.

Horseback riding as a therapy has been used for thousands of years. It was used in Greece in the fifth century B.C. to rehabilitate injured soldiers. Hippocrates wrote of horseback riding as a "natural exercise." Similarly, wounded soldiers were treated with horseback riding in England during World War I.

More recently, Liz Hartel, a Danish woman who had polio, demonstrated the possible benefits of riding. She developed leg strength and coordination through riding and eventually won a silver medal in dressage in the 1952 Olympic Games in Finland.

Riding therapy has been used since the 1940s in Europe, especially in Germany and Switzerland. Much of the published research in this area has been conducted in Germany. This type of therapy is a relative newcomer in the United States. The first center for therapeutic riding was established in Michigan in 1969. There are now more than 600 accredited therapeutic riding centers in the United States.

Treatment Method

Hippotherapy and therapeutic riding are often done in conjunction with physical therapy. In riding therapy, a person is placed on a horse and monitored by a therapist, usually a trained physical therapist or occupational therapist. Typically, bareback pads are used, and straps or handholds are provided for stability. In addition to the conventional riding position,

riders may also sit sideways or backwards or even lie sideways or backwards. The person on the horse responds to the animal's movements with
body movements. Unlike conventional horseback riding, in riding therapy, the rider does not attempt to control the horse. Rather, the therapist,
who may be on the ground or on the horse with the rider, controls the
horse and adjusts the treatment as indicated.

Studies in MS and Other Conditions

Hippotherapy is believed to be beneficial for people with walking difficulties because the rhythmic movements of the human pelvis while horseback
riding are similar to those that occur with walking. In addition, the variations in the horse's speed, stride, and direction are thought to be beneficial
for walking. Some studies indicate that approximately 100 different horse
movements are transmitted to the rider during each minute of riding.
There also may be some psychological benefits related to developing a
bond with the horse, developing relationships with the therapist and other
riders, and simply being outdoors.

Although hippotherapy is frequently discussed in relation to MS,
only a few studies have specifically evaluated its possible benefits for people with this disease. A preliminary study reported in 1988 examined the
effects of twice-weekly therapeutic riding for nine weeks in people with MS
(1). Riding was associated with improved walking and improved mood. In
another study reported in 1991, it was found that one person with MS had
a more normal walking pattern after once-weekly riding for four weeks (2).
Studies of hippotherapy indicate that it may have both physical and psy-
chosocial benefits. One recent preliminary study in Pennsylvania, reported
at an MS conference in May 1999, found that hippotherapy for six to eight
weeks improved balance and the quality of life in three people with MS.

Hippotherapy and therapeutic riding have been researched more
extensively in children with cerebral palsy. These studies are relevant to MS
because people with cerebral palsy and MS experience some of the same
neurologic difficulties, including walking unsteadiness, stiffness, and
weakness.

Unfortunately, many of the studies on cerebral palsy have been small
and poorly designed and have not included a placebo group. In addition,
inconsistent results have been obtained. In studies of once- or twice-weekly therapy, ranging from 8 to 26 weeks, therapy has been associated with
improvement in walking, running, jumping, muscle strength, and muscle
stiffness. In addition, one study found that children walked more efficient-

ly and used less energy to walk after therapy. Improvement in standing and sitting postures has also been associated with hippotherapy in some studies.

Studies have been done in other conditions. In a German study of people with significant arm or leg weakness, hippotherapy improved stiffness (spasticity), urinary function, bowel function, mood, and sleep. One study of children with language disorders reported improvement in language skills and self-esteem.

Although some studies have reported positive effects in MS, cerebral palsy, and other conditions, the results of these studies are not conclusive. Clearly, studies with larger numbers of patients and better design are needed to more fully understand the effects of this type of therapy.

Side Effects

The most obvious risk of hippotherapy and therapeutic horseback riding is falling from the horse! People with MS who are experiencing a significant exacerbation should probably avoid hippotherapy because they may be especially unstable. Also, riding may not be possible for people with severe muscle stiffness or spasticity. People with severe fatigue or symptoms worsened by heat should be cautious about riding in hot weather. The American Hippotherapy Association lists a number of other conditions that should preclude hippotherapy, including severe osteoporosis, bone fractures, herniated disks, instability of the spine, severe arthritis, the use of anticoagulant medication, wounds or sores on weight-bearing surfaces, and seizures. The Association also recommends that therapy be done cautiously with some conditions, including diabetes, hip joint abnormalities, obesity, mild or moderate osteoporosis, allergies to dust or horsehair, heart disease, incontinence, and recent surgery.

Practical Information

It is best to receive hippotherapy from a qualified therapist who works at a riding center. For those with mild disability, therapeutic riding sessions provide the benefits of riding as well as riding lessons. When the riding skills are learned, riding may be done independently.

Sessions generally last 20 to 30 minutes. Fees are approximately $35 to $150 per hour. Health insurance may cover some of the cost of the therapy.

More information on hippotherapy and therapeutic horseback riding may be obtained from:

- The American Hippotherapy Association, North American Riding for the Handicapped Association, P.O. Box 33150, Denver, Colorado 80233, 303-452-1212, or 800-369-RIDE
- The National Center for Equine Facilitated Therapy, 5001 Woodside Road, Woodside, California 94062, 650-851-2271

Conclusion

Hippotherapy and therapeutic horseback riding are low-risk, moderate-cost therapies that offer possible benefits for multiple MS-associated symptoms, including walking difficulties, spasticity, weakness, bladder and bowel problems, and depression. Further studies are needed to determine the effects of this therapy more definitively.

Additional Readings

Journal Articles

Bertoti DB. Effect of therapeutic horseback riding on posture in children with cerebral palsy. *Phys Ther* 1988; 68:1505–1512.

MacKinnon JR, Noh S, Lariviere J, et al. A study of therapeutic effects of horseback riding for children with cerebral palsy. *Phys Occup Ther Ped* 1995; 15:17–31.

MacKinnon Joyce R, Noh S, Laliberte D, et al. Therapeutic horseback riding: A review of the literature. *Phys Occup Ther Ped* 1995; 15:1–15.

McGibbon NH, Andrade C-K, Widener G, et al. Effect of an equine-movement therapy program on gait, energy expenditure, and motor function in children with spastic cerebral palsy: A pilot study. *Dev Med Child Neurol* 1998; 40:754–762.

Homeopathy

Homeopathy is one of the more controversial forms of CAM. Much of the controversy is due to the fact that the basic principles of homeopathy are in conflict with many of the fundamental concepts of conventional medicine as well as those of chemistry and physics. In spite of these controversial ideas, homeopathy is, on a worldwide basis, one of the most popular forms of CAM.

Homeopathy is a system of medicine that was developed in the 1800s by Samuel Hahnemann, a German physician. Homeopathy was very popular in Europe and North America in the nineteenth century. The use of homeopathy in the United States declined from the 1950s to the 1970s, but its popularity has rebounded since then.

Homeopathy is used globally. On a worldwide basis, $1 to 5 billion are spent yearly on this form of treatment. Homeopathy is most popular in Europe and India. Homeopathic remedies are dispensed in pharmacies in France, and 25 percent of German physicians use homeopathy in their clinical practice. In the United States, $227 million are spent on homeopathy on an annual basis. Homeopathy is growing by approximately 12 percent yearly in the United States, and approximately 1 percent of American adults currently use homeopathy.

Treatment Method

Homeopathy is based on several principles. One is the "law of similars," which states that "like cures like." Variations of this principle have been used in other forms of medicine for thousands of years. In homeopathy, it is believed that, if large doses of a substance produce specific symptoms, very small doses of that substance will cure the same symptoms. For example, because large doses of arsenic produce stomach cramps, very low doses of arsenic may be used to treat them.

The use of very low doses of substances is another important principle of homeopathy. Natural substances, such as herbs, minerals, or animal products, are mixed with water or alcohol and then diluted 1:10 or 1:100. These dilutions are then repeated many times such that the final solution is *extremely dilute*. In homeopathic notation, "X" is used for 1:10 dilutions, "C" is used for 1:100 dilutions, and a number is used for the number of times a specific dilution is made. For example, "12X" refers to a solution that has been diluted 12 times in a 1:10 manner, and "30C" signifies a 1:100 dilution performed 30 times.

Many homeopathic preparations are so dilute that they do not contain even a single molecule of the original substance. In this situation, it is argued that the water has a "memory" for the substance that it once contained. Also, by the laws of homeopathy, it is believed that a solution is *more* potent if it contains *less* of a substance. These ideas of water "memory" and increased potency with increased dilution, which defy the conventional laws of physics, chemistry, and biology, generate much of the controversy about homeopathy. The use of these dilute solutions has raised questions about whether homeopathy is simply a way to produce a placebo response.

Homeopathy is focused on identifying symptoms and the personal features of the individual. In addition, homeopathic treatment aims to use the body's natural healing processes. This is in contrast to conventional medicine in which symptoms are used primarily to diagnose an underlying disease; the personal characteristics of an individual are not a critical component of the diagnostic process or choice of therapy; and treatment involves the use of drugs and other therapies that improve the disease process but do not necessarily alter the body's natural healing abilities.

Because of the detailed evaluation process, homeopaths probably become more familiar with their patients and spend more time with them than do physicians who practice conventional medicine. One study found that physicians in the United States who practice homeopathy spend more than twice as much time with their patients than physicians who do not practice homeopathy. The in-depth relationship that develops in homeopathy may be important for the healing process and may certainly augment any type of placebo effect.

A variety of homeopathic remedies have been suggested for MS. The treatment regimen depends on the individual and the specific symptoms. Homeopathic remedies that are sometimes recommended for MS include *Argentum nitricum*, *Aurum muriaticum*, and *Plumbum metallicum*.

Could Homeopathy Be a Placebo Effect?

Because the approach of a homeopath may be conducive to a placebo effect and homeopathic remedies may not actually contain any active substance, much of the beneficial effect of homeopathy may be a placebo response. Even if it is a placebo response, it may be helpful in certain situations. It is known that placebos are generally 30 to 40 percent effective. For situations in which conventional medicine has no particularly effective therapy, homeopathy may be a way to provide at least a placebo response. Jeremy Swayne, an English homeopath, writes: "If homeopathy is placebo, it presents us with a rich and systematic study of the working of the placebo response, which fully deserves to be taken seriously and investigated. If it is not, then the implications are even more startling" (1).

Different Homeopathic Approaches

There are classic and nonclassic approaches in homeopathy. The classic approach involves a detailed evaluation by a practitioner who develops a personalized treatment plan on the basis of the clinical evaluation. In contrast, the nonclassic approach does not involve a homeopath. Instead, a certain condition is identified, and treatment for that condition is then given. In the nonclassic approach, the condition may be identified by the affected individual or by a nonhomeopath practitioner who uses homeopathic therapy.

Studies in MS and Other Conditions

Whether homeopathic therapy produces effects that are greater than those produced by placebos is subject to controversy. Many clinical studies have evaluated homeopathic treatment for a variety of conditions. Unfortunately, many of these studies have been poorly conducted, and the results are often not conclusive.

To attempt to clarify this area, two recent studies have evaluated the results of multiple homeopathic studies. In 1991, a report examined 107 homeopathic studies published between 1966 and 1990 (2). Most of the studies were of low quality. However, approximately three-fourths of them reported beneficial effects. A research article in 1997 analyzed the results of 89 homeopathic studies (3). This study concluded that no studies have clearly proven homeopathy to be an effective therapy for any specific condition. However, it was also argued in this study that the effects of homeopathy are not simply placebo effects. These studies indicate that future studies are necessary to determine the effectiveness of homeopathy.

Homeopathy is not one of the most commonly used forms of CAM among people with MS in the United States. In contrast, homeopathy is used frequently by people with MS in Europe. Recent studies have shown that among people with MS, homeopathy is the most popular form of CAM in Holland and one of the most popular CAM therapies in Germany.

Specific homeopathic remedies are sometimes recommended for MS. The medical literature contains isolated reports (anecdotes) of individuals with MS treated with homeopathy. However, there are no well-documented large studies of the effect of homeopathic treatment on MS.

The effects of homeopathy on other diseases have been investigated. Preliminary results indicate that homeopathy may improve symptoms in people with rheumatoid arthritis, which, like MS, is an autoimmune disorder. Homeopathy has produced mixed results for neurologic diseases other than MS. One low-quality study found that homeopathy was effective for anxiety and depression. Two studies in stroke found no benefit, while one preliminary study in people with mild head injury reported some positive effects. A beneficial response was found in one study of people with migraine headaches.

Viral infections, such as the common cold and flu, may lead to MS attacks. As a result, it may be helpful for people with MS to try to prevent viral infections or to shorten the time that they are affected by a viral infection. There are limited options for the treatment or prevention of viral infections, which include simple preventive measures (such as hand-washing and avoiding exposure to infected people), the flu vaccination, and recently developed prescription medications that decrease the duration and severity of the flu. Supplements of unproven effectiveness for the common cold (echinacea, garlic, zinc, vitamin C) pose a theoretical risk for people with MS because of possible immune-stimulating activity.

Given the limited options, some people consider the use of homeopathy for preventing or treating viral infections. Studies of homeopathic therapies for viral syndromes have produced mixed results. For people with an interest in homeopathic remedies, this approach may be a reasonable possibility for viral infections. If homeopathy is used, available conventional therapies should be discussed with a physician, and it must be kept in mind that the homeopathic therapies are not proven to be effective.

Side Effects

Overall, homeopathy is very well tolerated. Homeopathy should not be used in lieu of conventional medical therapy. Some of the substances used in homeopathy, such as snake venom, arsenic, and poison oak, are potentially toxic. However, the doses of these substances are generally so low that they do not cause problems.

Homeopaths note several precautions that should be taken. One is that treatment should stop when a symptom resolves. Otherwise, the treatment may produce recurrence of the symptom. Also, there are "antidotes" that may interfere with treatment. Antidotes include coffee, acupuncture, x-rays, and dental drilling. Finally, a person receiving homeopathic treatment should notify the homeopath of any conventional medical treatment that is being used because this information may affect the homeopathic interpretation of symptoms.

Practical Information

In choosing a homeopath, it is best to choose a practitioner who has graduated from a program accredited by the Council on Homeopathic Education. The five accredited programs are:

- Bastyr University, Seattle, Washington
- Hahnemann Medical Clinic, Albany, California
- International Foundation for Homeopathy, Seattle, Washington
- National College of Natural Health Sciences, Seattle, Washington
- Ontario College of Naturopathic Medicine, Toronto, Ontario

More information on homeopathy can be obtained from the National Center for Homeopathy (NCH) (http:// www.healthy.net/uch/nchsearch.htm); 801 North Fairfax Street, Suite 306, Alexandria, Virginia 22314 (703-548-7790).

Conclusion

Homeopathy is a low-risk, low–moderate cost therapy with unproven effectiveness. No rigorous studies have specifically evaluated the effect of homeopathy on MS. For people with MS who are interested in this approach, it may be worth considering for mild conditions (such as viral infections and low levels of pain or anxiety) or for conditions for which conventional medical therapy is ineffective or only partially effective. Homeopathy should not be used in place of conventional medicine. Specifically, homeopathic treatment should not be used for controlling MS disease activity in place of conventional medications such as Copaxone®, Avonex®, Betaseron®, and Rebif®.

Additional Readings

Books

Swayne J. *Homeopathic Method: Implications for Clinical Practice and Medical Science*. New York: Churchill Livingstone, 1998.

Journal Articles

Linde K, Clausius N, Ramirez G, et al. Are the clinical effects of homoeopathy placebo effects? A meta-analysis of placebo-controlled trials. *Lancet* 1997; 350:834–843.

Kleijnen J, Knipschild P, ter Riet G. Clinical trials of homoeopathy. *Br Med J* 1991; 302:316–326.

Hyperbaric Oxygen

Hyperbaric oxygen treatment is a form of oxygen therapy. It is claimed to be an effective treatment for a large number of diseases, including MS. Unfortunately, many of the claims about this therapy are not supported by research evidence.

Treatment Method

In this type of treatment, a person breathes oxygen under increased pressure in a specially designed chamber. The procedure increases the oxygen content of the blood and thereby increases the amount of oxygen in different body tissues. The increased oxygen level in the blood and tissues is believed to be helpful for a variety of medical conditions.

Studies in MS and Other Conditions

The study that stimulated interest in hyperbaric oxygen and MS was published in 1983 (1). In this study of 17 people with MS, 12 showed improvement and 5 had long-lasting improvement. In addition to this clinical study, animal studies have produced positive results. In animals, hyperbaric oxygen protects against EAE, an experimental form of MS.

Advocates of hyperbaric oxygen therapy for MS cite the positive clinical study from 1983. However, seven studies performed after the 1983 study did *not* demonstrate any consistent therapeutic effect for hyperbaric oxygen. In a few studies, there was a mild improvement in bladder problems. A 1995 review of hyperbaric oxygen treatment trials in MS concluded that hyperbaric oxygen did not produce significant benefits in MS and that this therapy should not be used for MS (2).

Hyperbaric oxygen is an accepted therapy for a limited number of specific medical conditions. For example, it is an effective treatment for burns and severe infections. Other rare uses included decompression sickness (as a result of deep-sea diving), carbon monoxide poisoning, air bubbles in the blood stream caused by medical procedures, and tissue injury caused by radiation exposure.

Side Effects

In general, hyperbaric oxygen is well tolerated. Mild and reversible visual changes may sometimes occur. Rarely, more serious side effects may occur, including seizures, pressure injury to the ear, cataracts, and collapsed lungs.

Practical Information

Hyperbaric oxygen therapy is time-consuming and expensive. Each session lasts from one to five hours, and a course of therapy may require 20 sessions. A course of treatment costs $10,000 to $20,000. It is costly because the equipment is expensive, technicians monitor the equipment during therapy, and many treatment sessions are usually involved.

Conclusion

There is no evidence to support the use of hyperbaric oxygen therapy in MS. Many studies have shown that it is not an effective treatment for MS. In addition, it is very expensive, requires much time and effort, and occasionally produces serious side effects.

Additional Readings

Journal Articles

Kleijnen J, Knipschild P. Hyperbaric oxygen for multiple sclerosis: Review of controlled trials. *Acta Neurol Scand* 1995; 91:330–334.

Tibbles PM, Edelsberg JS. Hyperbaric oxygen therapy. *N Engl J Med* 1996; 334:1642–1648.

Hypnosis and Guided Imagery

Hypnosis

Hypnosis uses mental processes to alter physical processes. In this way, hypnosis, like biofeedback and meditation, is a type of "mind–body therapy."

There has been medical interest in hypnosis for hundreds of years. In the late 1700s, Franz Mesmer, an Austrian physician, used calming gestures and words to relax patients and, presumably, to balance their magnetic energy. A commission appointed by the French Academy criticized this technique, known as mesmerism, and Mesmer was claimed to be a fraud. More recently, a magical, evil, mind-controlling view of hypnosis was promoted by vaudeville performers and magicians.

Hypnosis has gained some acceptance by conventional medicine despite these negative representations of the technique. It was deemed a valid medical treatment in England in 1955 and in the United States in 1958. Research studies support the use of hypnosis for some conditions. However, many physicians and other mainstream healthcare professionals do not readily incorporate hypnosis into their medical practices.

Treatment Method

In hypnosis, an individual enters a trancelike state. In this state of focused concentration, which is generally produced by a hypnotherapist, an individual is particularly vulnerable to suggestion. As a result, during hypnosis, a therapist makes suggestions with therapeutic value. For example, anxiety may be improved with suggestions of relaxation, and pain may be relieved with suggestions of numbness. In self-hypnosis, individuals make specific suggestions themselves. Self-hypnosis is usually most effective when it is taught by a trained therapist.

There is great variability in the success of hypnosis. Some of this variability is due to the fact that different people have different degrees of susceptibility to hypnotic suggestion. Approximately two-thirds of the population are moderately susceptible to suggestion, and 5 to 10 percent of people are extremely susceptible. Children and young adults are especially responsive to hypnosis.

Studies in MS and Other Conditions

No large studies have specifically evaluated the possible benefits of hypnosis for MS. However, symptoms that may occur with MS have been investigated in people with other conditions. Anxiety, which occurs frequently in MS, may be reduced through hypnosis-induced relaxation. Also, hypnosis may be an effective therapy for pain, which may be a particularly bothersome symptom in MS. Hypnosis appears to relieve different types of pain, including pain associated with surgery, breast cancer, and fibromyalgia, a rheumatologic condition. Hypnosis may be used during surgery to reduce the amount of anesthesia or to completely eliminate the need for anesthesia in some cases.

The effects of hypnosis on immune system function have been investigated in limited studies. Mixed results have been obtained in studies of immune function changes associated with hypnosis-induced relaxation. Hypnotic suggestions may be made to attempt to specifically alter immune function. In one study, four hypnotized individuals were given the suggestion to decrease their immunologic response to a skin test for tuberculosis; all of them inhibited this reaction.

Among neurologic disorders, some beneficial effects of hypnosis have been reported in people with migraine headaches, strokes, head injury, and spinal cord injury. Hypnosis has also been effective for some people with alcoholism, tobacco addiction, obesity, asthma, nausea and vomiting (resulting from cancer or pregnancy), and phobias.

Side Effects

Hypnosis is usually safe. Although some movies and television shows portray hypnotized individuals performing evil tasks, this is not an accurate view. People cannot be forced into hypnosis, and hypnotized people cannot be unwittingly instructed to commit undesirable acts. People with psychiatric disorders may experience adverse effects and should discuss their situation with a psychiatrist before considering hypnosis.

Practical Information

Several organizations provide information about hypnosis. One of these is The American Society of Clinical Hypnosis, 2200 East Devon Avenue, Suite 291, Des Plaines, Illinois 60018, 708-297-3317. Health insurance companies sometimes reimburse for hypnosis.

Conclusion

Hypnosis is a well-tolerated, low–moderate cost therapy. Although it has not been studied specifically in MS, hypnosis may relieve some MS-associated symptoms, including anxiety and pain.

Guided Imagery

Guided imagery is a technique frequently used in hypnosis as well as in meditation and other relaxation therapies. Although it is generally used to produce relaxation, guided imagery may be used for other purposes.

Treatment Method

In guided imagery, an individual creates images that have specific effects on the mind and the body. For example, to produce a state of relaxation, one may imagine sitting in a tranquil location such as a beach or a mountain. These images may be visual but may also involve sounds, taste, and smells associated with a particular setting.

Studies in MS and Other Conditions

Guided imagery has not undergone extensive investigation in MS. One study conducted in Pennsylvania evaluated the effects of imagery and relaxation techniques in 33 people with MS (1). For imagery, people were instructed to imagine repair of injured myelin and beneficial immune system activity. People who practiced daily imagery along with relaxation experienced less anxiety and produced more active and powerful images of their disease process. There was no effect of imagery and relaxation on depression or specific MS-associated symptoms. Other studies suggest that imagery improves anxiety and cancer- and surgery-related pain.

Imagery could conceivably be used to alter immune system function. Limited studies in this area have produced mixed results. In one study, people were instructed to use imagery to increase the adherence, or stickiness, of *neutrophils*, a specific type of immune cell (2). Each individual created his or her own image of neutrophil adherence. For example, one person envisioned ping-pong balls that exuded honey onto their surfaces and thereby adhered to all objects that they touched. The stickiness of the neutrophils increased in one of the groups that practiced imagery.

Guided imagery has been used for other conditions. Imagery is sometimes used to assist in managing heart disease because of its relaxation effect and ability to decrease blood pressure. Elite athletes use imagery to enhance athletic performance.

Side Effects

Imagery is generally well tolerated. It should not be used instead of conventional medication for serious conditions, such as modifying the course of MS. People with psychiatric conditions, including severe depression, should use caution with imagery. Also, imagery-induced relaxation may cause disturbing thoughts, fear of losing control, and anxiety.

Practical Information

Most imagery sessions last 20 to 30 minutes. Books and audiotapes are available for additional instruction. Alternatively, a trained therapist may be used. More information about guided imagery may be obtained from The Academy of Guided Imagery, P.O. Box 2070, Mill Valley, California 94942, 650-493-4430.

Conclusion

Guided imagery is inexpensive and safe. It may reduce anxiety and pain, but its therapeutic effects have not been fully investigated. Further studies are needed to examine its effectiveness.

Additional Readings

Books

Cassileth BR. *The Alternative Medicine Handbook.* New York: W.W. Norton, 1998:122–130.

Dillard J, Ziporyn T. *Alternative Medicine for Dummies.* Foster City, CA: IDG Books, 1998:197–203.

Fugh-Berman A. *Alternative Medicine: What Works.* Baltimore: Williams & Wilkins, 1997:139–146.

Journal Articles

Hall H, Minnes L, Olness K. The psychophysiology of voluntary immunomodulation. *Int J Neurosci* 1993; 69:221–234.

Maguire BL. The effects of imagery on attitudes and moods in multiple sclerosis patients. *Alt Ther* 1996; 2:75–79.

Smith GR, McKenzie JM, Marmer DJ, et al. Psychologic modulation of the human immune response to Varicella zoster. *Arch Intern Med* 1985; 145:221–235.

Van Fleet, S. Relaxation and imagery for symptom management: Improving patient assessment and individualizing treatment. ONF 2000; 27:501–510.

Magnets and Electromagnetic Therapy

The use of magnets and electromagnetic fields is a type of "energy medicine." Magnets and electricity have been used for medicinal purposes for thousands of years. They were used in ancient China to stimulate acupuncture sites. In the eleventh and twelfth centuries, it was claimed that lodestones, minerals with natural magnetic qualities, relieved a variety of medical conditions. Paracelsus, a sixteenth century Swiss physician and alchemist, used magnets to treat seizures. In the eighteenth century, Franz Mesmer, an Austrian physician, proposed a theory of "animal magnetism" and wrote a book on the subject, *On the Medicinal Uses of the Magnet*. It was later found that his therapy was based on hypnotism (see section in this book), not on any therapeutic effects of magnets. A large number of magnetic and electrical devices were promoted during the nineteenth century, the "golden age of medical electricity." These devices included magnetic insoles, belts, girdles, and caps. The manufacture and sale of magnetic devices in the United States is now limited by the Food, Drug and Cosmetic Act and the Medical Devices Amendment of 1976. Several recent research studies on magnets have increased interest in this type of therapy.

Treatment Method

Magnets and electricity are used in both conventional and unconventional medicine. In conventional medicine, small amounts of electrical energy produced by the body are measured for diagnostic reasons. For example, an electroencephalogram (EEG) records electrical energy produced by the brain, whereas an electrocardiogram (ECG or EKG) detects electrical currents produced by the heart. Magnetic resonance imaging (MRI) machines use very powerful magnets to produce images of different parts of the body.

A unique therapeutic use of electrical energy has been employed recently to treat tremors in people with MS, Parkinson's disease, and other neurologic disorders. In this treatment, which is under active investigation, an electrode is implanted in a brain region involved in controlling body movements. Electrical stimulation of the electrode may significantly improve the tremor.

There are many unconventional uses of magnets and electricity. Two types of electromagnetic therapy are usually considered for MS. One type of therapy uses magnets that are available as bracelets, belts, and even large mats that may be placed on a bed. The other form of therapy uses devices that produce pulsing weak electromagnetic fields. It is claimed that magnet therapy and pulsing electromagnetic therapy produce beneficial effects by correcting disease-causing electrical imbalances in the body.

Studies in MS and Other Conditions

A promising two-part study of electromagnetic therapy in people with MS was reported from Hungary in 1987 (1). In the first part of this study, which included the use of a placebo therapy, 70 to 80 percent of the 20 treated participants benefited from pulsed electromagnetic therapy applied to the spine and legs. Spasticity, pain, and bladder function improved. In the second part of the investigation, electromagnetic treatment was used in 104 people in a less rigorous manner. Once again, symptoms improved in approximately 80 percent of people.

There are two other studies of electromagnetic therapy in MS. In 1996, a Danish group published a report on pulsing electromagnetic therapy applied to the spine in 38 people with MS (2). This study, which focused on spasticity, found a significant reduction in spasticity with electromagnetic therapy. In 1997, a placebo-controlled study from the University of Washington examined the effects of a pulsing device applied to three acupuncture points on 30 people with MS (3). Benefits were noted with spasticity, bladder function, cognitive problems, fatigue, mobility, and vision. In addition to these studies of large groups of people with MS, there are reports of individuals with MS who experienced improvement in multiple symptoms with electromagnetic therapy.

Magnets have been investigated in other conditions. Among neurologic disorders, small studies have found that magnet therapy may be beneficial for people with pain associated with the delayed effects of polio (post-polio syndrome) and for people with pain resulting from nerve injury related to diabetes and other conditions. Magnets do not appear to be effective for treating long-standing low back pain.

Pulsing electromagnetic therapy may have multiple applications. This type of therapy stimulates healing of bone fractures. It may also decrease swelling resulting from ankle sprains, promote healing of bed-sores, and improve joint mobility and pain in people with arthritis.

Magnets are not approved by the FDA for any medical condition at this time. However, pulsing devices are approved by the FDA for the treatment of bone fractures that do not heal. These devices have been used by more than 200,000 people.

A fascinating area of research involves applying pulsing high-intensity magnetic fields to the scalp. This technique, known as transcranial magnetic stimulation, takes advantage of the ability of magnetic fields to pass through bone. In this procedure, a very strong magnetic field applied to the scalp passes through the skull and stimulates the underlying brain tissue. For example, applying magnetic stimulation to the region of the brain that controls movement results in movement of the corresponding part of the body. Some studies indicate that this therapy may be effective for depression and anxiety. Further studies are needed to determine the effectiveness and long-term safety of this technique. This approach is only available in designated research centers because very strong magnetic fields are used.

Side Effects

The use of magnets and pulsing electromagnetic fields is generally well tolerated, but the long-term safety of these therapies is not known. Women who are pregnant and people with pacemakers and other implanted electronic medical devices should consult a physician before using this type of therapy. High-intensity magnetic fields may have significant side effects (headaches, hearing loss, seizures, and other possible unknown effects) and should only be used under the direction of qualified clinical investigators.

Practical Information

A large number of magnets and pulsing electromagnetic devices are available. These vary greatly in terms of strength, size, shape, composition, and cost. Although some companies claim that their products are better because they produce a stronger electromagnetic field, it is not clear that a stronger field necessarily provides more benefit.

Conclusion

The use of low-intensity magnets and pulsing electromagnetic fields is usually well tolerated. Several studies suggest that pulsing electromagnetic fields may improve multiple MS symptoms, especially spasticity and bladder function. Other symptoms that may benefit from this therapy are fatigue, pain, cognitive problems, and walking. Further studies are required to definitely determine whether electromagnetic therapy in MS is effective and safe.

Additional Readings

Books

Cassileth BR. *The Alternative Medicine Handbook.* New York: W.W. Norton, 1998:299–304.

Fugh-Berman A. *Alternative Medicine: What Works.* Baltimore: Williams & Wilkins, 1997:189–191.

Journal Articles

Guseo A. Pulsing electromagnetic field therapy of multiple sclerosis by the Gyuling-Bordas device: Double-blind, cross-over and open studies. *J Bioelec* 1987; 6:23–35.

Nielsen JF, Sinkjaer T, Jakobsen J. Treatment of spasticity with repetitive magnetic stimulation: A double-blind placebo-controlled study. *Multiple Sclerosis* 1996; 2:227–232.

George MS, Lisanby SAH, Sackeim HA. Transcranial magnetic stimulation: Applications in neuropsychiatry. *Arch Gen Psych* 1999; 56:300–311.

Richards TL, Lappin MS, Acosta-Urquidi J, et al. Double-blind study of pulsing magnetic field effects on multiple sclerosis. *J Alt Complem Med* 1997; 3:21–29.

Vallbona C, Hazlewood CF, Jurida G. Response of pain to static magnetic fields in postpolio patients: A double-blind pilot study. *Arch Phys Med Rehabil* 1997; 78:1200–1203.

~Marijuana

~Marijuana is derived from the plant known as *Cannabis sativa*, one of the oldest cultivated plants. It was grown in China nearly 5,000 years ago and has been used medicinally in many different cultures for thousands of years.

Treatment Method

There are several forms of marijuana. The main active constituent in marijuana, a chemical known as Δ9-tetrahydrocannabinol or THC, is available by prescription as a pill (dronabinol or Marinol®). A synthetic form of THC (nabilone or Cesamet®) is also available as a pill in Canada, Europe, and Australia. Most simply, the leaf may be smoked.

Studies in MS and Other Conditions

The effects of marijuana, THC, and nabilone have been studied in many diseases, including MS. On March 17, 1999, the National Academy of Sciences/Institute of Medicine (NAS/IOM) released a report that analyzed the scientific and clinical literature on potential beneficial effects of marijuana. The NAS/IOM report concluded that marijuana or THC may be effective in the treatment of pain, nausea associated with chemotherapy, and weight loss associated with AIDS and cancer. The report also cautioned against the long-term use of smoked marijuana, indicated that effective prescription medications are available for many conditions treated with marijuana, and suggested that methods of taking the drug other than smoking it should be developed.

The NAS/IOM analysis indicated that there have been some positive studies of marijuana and THC in relieving spasticity, or muscle stiffness, associated with MS. These studies have been of mixed quality in that they have involved small numbers of patients (sometimes only one patient) and have not been well-designed clinical trials. Despite these limitations, there have been promising reports of marijuana, THC, or nabilone decreasing spasticity. These studies have not compared this treatment effect with that of prescription drugs for spasticity. Further studies with better design and more patients are needed to clarify the effects of these compounds on spasticity and other MS-related symptoms.

In January 1999, the United Nations and the Royal Pharmaceutical Society in the United Kingdom began enrolling people with MS in a study of marijuana and spasticity. This large study will evaluate the effects of THC or cannabis oil on spasticity in 300 to 400 people with MS.

A small study evaluated the effects of marijuana on a different MS symptom known as *nystagmus*, a jerking or twitching of eye movements (1). In this study of only one person, smoking marijuana reduced the severity of the nystagmus. This effect was consistently observed on three separate occasions, and the decrease in nystagmus occurred when there was an increase in the blood levels of cannabinoids, which are marijuana-derived chemicals. Interestingly, there was no effect with nabilone or capsules containing cannabis oil.

Studies of marijuana and THC effects on MS-associated gait unsteadiness have shown either no benefit or a worsening of this symptom. Minimal changes have been observed in limited studies on tremor in people with MS. The effects of marijuana on MS-associated pain have not been investigated in a clinical study.

In 1997, a survey of marijuana use in people with MS was reported (2). This study was conducted in the United States and the United Kingdom. A survey such as this is very different from a formal clinical study because people are not evaluated by objective test measures. Rather, people simply give their own assessment, and consequently the results are less reliable. In this survey, relief of spasticity was the most common benefit of marijuana and was reported by 97 percent of the respondents. Improvement of pain and tremor was reported by more than 90 percent. People had used marijuana for an average of six years. The frequency of marijuana use was remarkable; on average, it was used nearly three times per day and six days per week.

The effects of marijuana-derived chemicals on MS symptoms have been investigated in animals. In one study, mice with EAE, an experimental form of MS, exhibited spasticity and tremor (3). Interestingly, THC and two other marijuana-derived chemicals reduced both spasticity and tremor in these animals.

At this time, human studies of marijuana have evaluated MS-associated symptoms, such as spasticity or tremor. The effects of marijuana on

MS itself have not been investigated in human clinical studies. It is interesting to note that both animal and human studies have shown that marijuana and THC suppress the immune system. It is conceivable that this immune-suppressing effect is beneficial for MS. In EAE, an animal model of MS, several studies demonstrate that treatment with THC or THC-related compounds decreases the injury to the brain tissue and reduces the severity of the neurologic symptoms. Although these animal studies are promising, human studies need to be conducted to determine whether such a beneficial effect occurs in people with MS.

Side Effects

Smoking marijuana has significant adverse effects. First, there is a risk of cancer. Marijuana smoke contains known cancer-causing compounds, including nitrosamine and benzene, and it has been estimated that marijuana smoke contains 50 percent more cancer-causing chemicals than tobacco smoke. One study found that marijuana smoking was associated with a two- to threefold increased risk of developing cancer in the head and neck region, including the mouth, tongue, and throat.

Other risks are related to marijuana smoking. Marijuana use may damage the lungs, increase the risk of heart attack, and lead to poor outcomes with pregnancy. Neurologically, marijuana may increase the risk of seizures and may produce memory difficulties, confusion, incoordination, and weakness. How marijuana interacts with other drugs, particularly those that are used frequently in MS, is not known. Marijuana may increase the sedating effects of medications. One case of mania, or excessive arousal and excitability, occurred when marijuana was taken in combination with fluoxetine (Prozac®). Finally, *marijuana use is illegal in many states and countries.*

Conclusion

Research studies suggest that marijuana may decrease MS-associated spasticity. However, marijuana use is associated with significant side effects, and the possible interactions of marijuana with prescription medications are not well understood. Further research on the use of marijuana and marijuana-related chemicals is needed. If marijuana is used for MS symptoms, the user should discuss this use with a physician and should be aware that marijuana use may be illegal and that prescription medications for MS symptoms may be more effective and safer than marijuana.

Additional Readings

Books

Iversen LL. *The Science of Marijuana*. New York: Oxford University Press, 2000.

Nahas GG (ed.). *Marihuana and Medicine*. Totowa, NJ: Humana Press, 1999.

Journal Articles

Baker D, Pryce G, Croxford J, et al. Cannabinoids control spasticity and tremor in a multiple sclerosis model. *Nature* 2000; 404:84–87.

Consroe P, Musty R, Rein J, et al. The perceived effects of smoked cannabis on patients with multiple sclerosis. *Eur Neurol* 1997; 38:44–48.

Levy B. U.S. and U.N. studies support medicinal marijuana research. *Herbal Gram* 1999; 46:14–15.

Meinck HM, Schonle PW, Conrad B. Effect of cannabinoids on spasticity and ataxia in multiple sclerosis. *J Neurol* 1989; 236:120–122.

Mitka M. Therapeutic marijuana use supported while thorough proposed study done. *JAMA* 1999; 281:1473–1474.

Ungerleider JT, Andyrsiak T, Fairbanks L, et al. Delta-9-THC in the treatment of spasticity associated with multiple sclerosis. *Adv Alc Subst Abuse* 1987; 7:39–50.

Wirguin I, Mechoulam R, Breuer A, et al. Suppression of experimental autoimmune encephalomyelitis by cannabinoids. *Immunopharmacology* 1994; 28:209–214.

Massage

*M*assage is a healing method that has been used for thousands of years. It was a recommended therapy in ancient China and Egypt. Many common forms of massage now used in the United States are derived from Swedish massage, which was developed by a Swedish physician in the nineteenth century. Massage may be provided on its own or may be a component of other forms of alternative healing, including Ayurveda, traditional Chinese medicine, and aromatherapy.

Treatment Method

Massage is usually done on a specially designed table in a warm, quiet room with soft lighting and relaxing music. The individual receiving the massage is partially or completely undressed; a sheet or towel is used to cover parts of the body that are not being massaged. The therapist uses a variety of techniques, including pressing, stroking, rubbing, slapping, and tapping. Oil or lotion is usually used to make the movements smoother.

There are several possible mechanisms by which massage may be effective. First, massage appears to relax muscles (although only limited studies have formally evaluated this effect). This effect may be helpful for conditions that are worsened by muscle stiffness, such as headaches, neck pain, and low back pain. Also, massage may release chemicals known as *endorphins*, which reduce pain. Through a theoretical process known as "gate control," which presumes that only a certain number of impulses may reach the brain from a specific body part, stimulation by massage in a painful area may decrease the number of pain impulses received by the brain from that area. Finally, the simple act of touching that occurs with massage may convey positive feelings that are difficult to evaluate rigorously, such as caring, comfort, and acceptance. Touching is a simple and possibly beneficial act that is often missing from interactions with physicians and other mainstream healthcare providers.

Studies in MS and Other Conditions

Few studies have specifically evaluated massage therapy in people with MS. In a study reported in 1998, 24 people with MS who received massage therapy were compared with those who did not (1). In this small study, massage therapy was associated with multiple benefits, including increased self-esteem, improved social functioning, and reduced anxiety and depression. In addition, the group that received massage had better images of their bodies and the progression of their disease.

Symptoms that may occur with MS have been studied in other conditions. However, nearly all these studies have serious limitations, and consequently the results must not be taken as definitive. Some studies have shown a reduction in stress, anxiety, and depression. It is often stated that spasticity, or stiffness in the arms or legs, may improve with massage; studies in this area are surprisingly limited. Headache, low back pain, and other forms of pain, all of which may occur with MS, have responded to massage in some research studies. Cancer-related pain may improve with massage, and the National Cancer Institute recognizes massage as a nonmedication therapy for pain.

In addition to its effects on specific symptoms, massage may also have a beneficial effect on self-esteem and overall quality of life through its "healing touch" properties. Dr. Elizabeth Forsythe, an English physician with MS, wrote about her experiences with massage in the book *Multiple Sclerosis: Exploring Sickness and Health*: "Her patience, acceptance, and her remarkable hands began to lessen my loathing for my body. The massage also relieved much of the muscle spasm and tension in my body. Being massaged by somebody known and trusted is a good start to the building or rebuilding of a personal world of trust" (2).

The effects of massage on the immune system are not well understood. Immune stimulation has been reported with massage, but the significance of this effect is not known. In one study, infants with AIDS, an immune deficiency state, were treated with massage and had a better course than those who did not receive massage.

Side Effects

Massage is usually well tolerated. Minor adverse effects that have been reported include headache, muscle pain, and lethargy. There are also rare, isolated reports of more serious complications, such as bleeding into the liver with deep abdominal massage.

To prevent complications, there are certain conditions in which massage should be avoided or practiced with caution. The following guidelines should be followed:

■ Recent injuries should not be massaged.

■ Abdominal massage should be avoided by people with ulcers or enlargement of the liver or spleen.

■ People with fever, infection, clotted blood vessels (thrombosis), and jaundice should avoid massage.

■ Those with cancer, arthritis, and heart disease should consult a physician before receiving massage therapy.

■ Women who are pregnant should only receive massage from therapists who are experienced in pregnancy massage.

Practical Information

Massage is often performed by a therapist, but it may also be done on one's own without a therapist. Massage therapy sessions typically last from 30 to 90 minutes and cost $30 to $60 per hour. The expense of massage therapy is covered by some insurance plans. You can locate a massage therapist in the yellow pages of the telephone book.

More information about massage and qualified massage therapists is available from:

■ The American Massage Therapy Association, 820 Davis Street, Suite 100, Evanston Illinois, 60201, 312-761-2682

■ National Certification Board for Therapeutic Massage and Bodywork, 8201 Greensboro Drive, Suite 300, McLean, Virginia 22102, 800-296-0664 or 703-610-9015

Conclusion

Massage is a relatively safe, low–moderate cost therapy that may have several benefits. Although it has not been extensively studied in MS, limited studies in other conditions suggest that it may be helpful for some MS-associated symptoms, including anxiety, depression, muscle stiffness (spasticity), low back pain, and other types of pain.

Additional Readings

Books

Dillard J, Ziporyn T. *Alternative Medicine for Dummies*. Foster City, CA: IDG Books, 1998:161–180.
Fugh-Berman A. *Alternative Medicine: What Works*. Baltimore: Williams & Wilkins, 1997:147–157.
Vickers A. *Massage and Aromatherapy: A Guide for Health Professionals*. London: Chapman & Hall, 1996.

Journal Articles

Hernandez-Reif M, Field T, Field T, et al. Multiple sclerosis patients benefit from massage therapy. *J Bodywork Movement Ther* 1998; 2:168–174.

Meditation

Meditation is a type of "mind–body therapy," a class of therapies that also includes biofeedback, hypnosis, and guided imagery. Meditation has been practiced in some form for thousands of years, especially in the context of religious practice. Also, meditation is one of several components of some CAM therapies, including Ayurveda ("transcendental meditation," or TM) and traditional Chinese medicine.

Meditation is a way of producing the "relaxation response," which has been described extensively by Dr. Herbert Benson at the Harvard Medical School and The Mind/Body Medical Institute. The relaxation response is a state of relaxation that is associated with decreased anxiety, muscle relaxation, and lowering of blood pressure. It is believed to be the opposite of the physiologic response known as the "fight-or-flight response," characterized by the activation or stimulation of multiple body processes, such as increases in heart rate, blood pressure, and breathing rate.

Treatment Method

There are many different meditation methods. All of these techniques elicit relaxation by focusing concentration, relaxing the body, and diverting attention from stressful thoughts and feelings. One of the simplest strategies is outlined by Dr. Herbert Benson in *The Relaxation Response:*

1. Sit in a comfortable position in a quiet room and close your eyes.
2. Relax your muscles by starting with the feet and slowly working up the body to the face.
3. Each time you exhale, say a word silently.
4. Try to avoid distracting thoughts.
5. Continue this process for 10 to 20 minutes.

Other, more formal, meditation methods include transcendental meditation, mindfulness meditation (or vipassana), and meditation techniques associated with Zen (the Chinese word for meditation) and yoga. The relaxation response may also be produced by hypnosis, guided imagery, biofeedback, and prayer, all of which are discussed in detail elsewhere in this book.

Studies in MS and Other Conditions

No studies have formally evaluated the effects of meditation in a large number of people with MS. In one study of 40 people, 9 of whom had MS, meditation along with imagery decreased both anxiety and physical complaints during the physical rehabilitation process (1).

Other research studies have examined meditation effects on symptoms that may occur with MS but have involved people with conditions other than MS. It has been found that meditation may improve stress, anxiety, depression, and various types of pain, including low back pain and pain that occurs after surgery. Although difficult to study formally, feelings of control, empowerment, and self-esteem may develop through meditation. *Progressive muscle relaxation*, a specific process sometimes used in meditation, may improve insomnia.

Interestingly, meditation and other relaxation methods may produce changes in immune function. Various immune system changes have been described. The precise effects and their impact on MS are not fully understood at this time.

An interesting example of the influence of meditation on immune function was described in a 1985 report (2). A woman experienced in an Eastern religious–type of meditation was given small skin injections of a component of the chickenpox virus. Because she had been exposed to the virus previously, she had, as expected, an immune response to the injection that involved inflammation and redness of skin. Subsequently, she was told to use her meditation skills to attempt to decrease the injection response for a three-week period. For each week during that time, her skin reaction was reduced and the activity of her immune cells was decreased.

Meditation has been investigated in a number of other medical conditions. It may improve psoriasis (a skin condition), decrease seizure frequency, reduce blood pressure, and improve heart function in people with heart disease. Meditation has also produced some beneficial results in studies of heroin, cocaine, and nicotine addiction.

Side Effects

Meditation does not usually involve any serious risks. It may produce difficulties in people with serious psychiatric diseases, such as severe depression and schizophrenia. The state of relaxation elicited by meditation may produce fear of losing control, disturbing thoughts, and anxiety. Meditation should not be used in place of conventional therapy to treat MS or serious MS-associated symptoms.

Practical Information

Meditation may be done independently by following techniques described in books such as *The Relaxation Response* (see preceding). Classes in meditation techniques are often available through hospitals, health clubs, and community centers. If meditation is pursued, it is important to keep in mind that it often does not have immediate effects. It may take several weeks or months of practice to achieve significant relaxation.

Conclusion

Meditation is a well-tolerated, low-cost therapy that may provide medical benefits without the use of medication. For people with MS, meditation may be helpful for relieving stress, anxiety, depression, insomnia, and pain. It may also improve self-esteem and feelings of control.

Additional Readings

Books

Benson H. *The Relaxation Response*. New York: Avon Books, 1976.
Dillard J, Ziporyn T. Alternative Medicine for Dummies. Foster City, CA: IDG Books, 1998:187–196.
Fugh-Berman A. *Alternative Medicine: What Works*. Baltimore: Williams & Wilkins, 1997:167–174.

Journal Articles

Smith GR, McKenzie JM, Marmer DJ, et al. Psychologic modulation of the human immune response to Varicella Zoster. *Arch Int Med* 1985; 145:2110–2112.
Zachariae R, Kristensen JS, Hokland P, et al. Effect of psychological intervention in the form of relaxation and guided imagery on cellular immune function in normal healthy subjects: An overview. *Psychother Psychosom* 1990; 54:32–39.

Music Therapy

As its name implies, music therapy uses music to facilitate healing. This type of therapy has been practiced for thousands of years. It was used in some form in ancient Egypt and ancient Greece. Singing and drumming are also components of shamanic and Native American healing.

In the United States, music therapy degrees were first granted in the 1940s. Conventional medicine has increasingly recognized music therapy over the past decade. In 1992, the United States Congress approved a $1 million dollar yearly budget for research and education on music therapy in elderly people. There are currently more than 5,000 music therapists in the United States.

Treatment Method

In music therapy, people either create or listen to music. The appropriate form of therapy for a specific person is determined by a trained music therapist. Music therapy may be practiced on an individual basis or a group basis. Music is also sometimes used to facilitate imagery (see "Hypnosis and Guided Imagery").

The mechanism by which music therapy may work is not known. Some of its benefits may be related to music-induced relaxation. In addition, for people with movement difficulties such as incoordination or walking disorders, music therapy may elicit "entrainment," which essentially means that moving to the music makes movements more rhythmic, regular, and efficient.

Studies in MS and Other Conditions

Music therapy has undergone limited investigation. It has been studied for symptoms that may occur with MS. In general, these have been small clinical studies, and the conclusions therefore are not definitive.

155

Music therapy may have emotional and cognitive benefits. It has been shown to decrease anxiety in adults with heart disease and strokes and in children and adults undergoing surgery. Limited studies suggest that music therapy improves depression and decreases agitation and aggression in people with Alzheimer's disease. Music also appears to improve cognitive function. It may facilitate learning in children and college students and may improve attention and concentration in people with Alzheimer's disease.

Physical symptoms may benefit from music therapy. Music therapy has been beneficial for walking unsteadiness and incoordination in children and in adults with stroke and Parkinson's disease. It also lessens the effects of pain associated with labor, cancer, arthritis, and medical and dental procedures.

Side Effects

Music therapy is essentially risk-free, although excessive noise (greater than 90 decibels) may impair hearing and increase blood pressure.

Practical Information

More information about music therapy and qualified music therapists may be obtained from The American Music Therapy Association, 8455 Colesville Road, Suite 1000, Silver Spring Maryland, 20910, 301-589-3300, http://www.musictherapy.org.

Conclusion

Music therapy is a safe and inexpensive approach that may be beneficial for some MS symptoms. Although there are no large studies in people with MS, studies in other groups of people suggest that music therapy may be helpful for anxiety, depression, cognitive problems, walking difficulties, incoordination, and pain. Further research of its effectiveness is needed.

Additional Readings

Books

Gaynor ML. *Sounds of Healing: A Physician Reveals the Therapeutic Power of Sounds, Voice, and Music.* New York: Broadway Books, 1999.

Journal Articles

Cunningham MF, Monson B, Bookbinder MA. Introducing a music program in the perioperative area. *ORN J* 1997; 66:674–682.

Kneafsey R. The therapeutic use of music in a care of the elderly setting: A literature review. *J Clin Nurs* 1997; 6:341–346.

Marwick C. Music therapists chime in with data on medical results. *JAMA* 2000; 283:731–733.

Neuralyn

Neuralyn is a compound that is claimed to be effective for treating MS and many other diseases. It was developed by the Alternative Medicine and Biophysics Research Institute in Nampa, Idaho.

Treatment Method

According to information from the company, Neuralyn is a dilute solution of natural extracts, vitamins, and amino acids. It is administered through the skin.

The mechanism by which Neuralyn might produce its effects is not clear. Literature on the product states that it has many different biological effects, including muscle relaxation, improved metabolism, decreased inflammation, and pain relief. It is claimed to have effects on the central nervous system.

Studies in MS and Other Conditions

Based on literature from the company, Neuralyn is reported to be 85 percent effective for MS. Although there are anecdotal reports of people with MS improving with Neuralyn therapy, there are no large published clinical studies of Neuralyn treatment for MS. It is claimed that Neuralyn is very effective for other neurologic conditions, including migraines, spinal cord injury, Parkinson's disease, "paralysis," and pain. It is also recommended for cancer and "therapy-resistant illness."

Practical Information

According to 1999 information from the Alternative Medicine and Biophysics Research Institute, Neuralyn is administered in two-week intensive sessions, with four of these sessions scheduled over the course of the next 11 to 24 months. The cost is significant. Based on the company's information, four treatment sessions and yearly follow-up visits cost approximately $10,000.

Side Effects

According to the company, Neuralyn does not have any side effects and does not interact with any other medications.

Conclusion

No large published studies have evaluated the safety or effectiveness of Neuralyn treatment for MS. In addition, the treatment is expensive and the scientific rationale for its use in MS is not clear. At this time, there is not strong evidence to support the use of Neuralyn for MS.

Pets

*P*ets are not necessarily a form of CAM. Caring for a pet may be considered a component of one's lifestyle or a hobby. However, caring for a pet may provide health benefits for people with MS and other medical conditions and usually is not considered in the context of a regular medical visit.

Pets are a part of everyday life for many people, but they may provide special benefits for people with medical conditions. The concept that pets may be therapeutic is not new. In the nineteenth century, the nurse Florence Nightingale, who loved pets and had exotic pets of her own, wrote: "A small pet animal is often an excellent companion for the sick . . ." (1). Recently, pets have been used increasingly in medical settings, and studies indicate that they provide health benefits.

Pets may improve both physical and emotional disorders. For people with physical disabilities, trained pets, especially dogs, assist by performing physical tasks, such as retrieving items or by stabilizing people who have walking difficulties. Pets are also sometimes used to assist people with physical rehabilitation, which may involve physical, occupational, or speech therapy.

Emotionally, it has been claimed that pets provide "unconditional love"; they are accepting and noncritical companions. Pets have been associated with relaxation and improvement in depression. They may also improve self-esteem and increase independence, responsibility, and companionship. Pets are sometimes brought into the hospital to provide possible psychological benefits for children.

Studies in MS and Other Conditions

Clinical studies of pets are limited. There are no large, well-designed studies of pets in people with MS. In the elderly, pets appear to improve many quality of life measures, including mental function, mood, life satisfaction, and psychological well-being. Pets may increase survival in people with heart disease. For people with high blood pressure, pets may minimize the increase in blood pressure that occurs in stressful situations.

Side Effects

Pets are generally well tolerated. However, some considerations should be kept in mind. Obviously, people with allergies should avoid pets that provoke allergies, and people who feel uncomfortable or stressed around pets probably would not benefit from their presence. Adequate care and an appropriate amount of space should be provided. Finally, pets should not substitute for basic emotional needs that should be obtained from humans. They may be used for a certain level of companionship, but this should not lead to social isolation.

Practical Information

More information on pets can be obtained from:

- Canine Companions for Independence, P.O. Box 446, Santa Rosa, California 95402, 800-572-2275, http://www.caninecompanions.org.
- Delta Society, P.O. Box 1080, Renton, Washington 98057, 800-869-6898, http://www.petsforum.com\\deltasociety
- Independence Dogs, Inc., 146 Stateline Road, Chaddsford, Pennsylvania 19317, 610-358-2723, http://www.ndepot.com\\idi.

Conclusion

Caring for a pet is a low-risk, low–moderate cost activity that may provide some psychological benefits. Trained pets may be helpful to people with weakness, clumsiness, or walking difficulties.

Additional Readings

Journal Articles

Doskoch P (ed.). A neurologic patient's best friend? Neurol Rev 1998; 13–14.
Dossey L. The healing power of pets: A look at animal-assisted therapy. Alt Ther 1997; 3:8–16.

The Pilates Method and the Physicalmind Method

The Pilates method and a variant of Pilates, the Physicalmind method, are two types of bodywork that are intended to increase flexibility and strength. The Pilates method was created during World War I by Joseph H. Pilates, a German inventor, boxer, and dancer. He developed the technique to help soldiers recover from war injuries. Pilates has been practiced in the United States since the 1920s, and its popularity grew significantly in the 1990s.

In the Pilates method, individuals concentrate on body movements. During exercises, which include more than 500 specific movements, attention is focused on which muscles are used and how they are controlled. There also is an emphasis on deep, coordinated breathing. The Physicalmind method was developed in response to a lawsuit regarding the Pilates name. In this spin-off of the original technique, there is more focus on the position of the body. Both the Pilates method and the Physicalmind method require the use of specialized exercise equipment.

Both methods are claimed to have several beneficial effects. They are supposed to improve strength and flexibility without increasing the size of muscles. Consequently, these methods are particularly popular among dancers.

Studies in MS and Other Conditions

There are no large clinical studies of the Pilates method or the Physicalmind method. Most claims of benefit from these therapies are based on anecdotes. Although both methods are used by some people with MS, these techniques have not been specifically investigated in this disease. In one of the few published studies of this therapy, six elite gymnasts at the

162

University of Illinois received one month of leap training combined with the Pilates method and pool training (1). This training regimen resulted in an increased height of jumps, improved reaction times, and increased strength. Clearly, further studies of the effectiveness of the Pilates method and the Physicalmind method are needed.

Side Effects

It is generally assumed that the Pilates method and the Physicalmind method are well tolerated.

Practical Information

The Pilates method and the Physicalmind method are taught either individually or in small groups. The techniques should be learned from a trained and certified instructor. The exercises may be done individually after receiving training. Adequate training usually requires a total of 20 to 30 sessions; each session generally costs $30 to $70. More information may be obtained from The Pilates Studio, 2121 Broadway, Suite 201, New York, NY, 800-474-5283, www.pilates-studio.com.

Conclusion

The Pilates method and the Physicalmind method are low-risk, moderate-cost forms of bodywork. These therapies are claimed to improve strength and flexibility, but there are few published studies that have evaluated their effectiveness.

Additional Readings

Journal Articles

Anonymous. Conditioning by Pilates. *Harvard Women's Health Watch* 1999; 6:7.
Hutchinson MR, Tremain L, Christiansen J, et al. Improving leaping ability in elite rhythmic gymnasts. *Med Sci Sports Ex* 1998; 30:1543–1547.

Prayer and Spirituality

Religion has been a fundamental aspect of human culture for tens of thousands of years. Recent surveys in the United States indicate that nearly 90 percent of the general population believe that there is a God who responds to prayer. Also, nearly 80 percent of the general population and 75 percent of physicians believe that spiritual faith can improve recovery from a disease.

The term *spirituality* refers to devotion to religious values. Prayer is a component of religious practice that may be used to give thanks to or obtain help from a higher power. Prayer is used to attempt to influence processes and events that are beyond human control, including health and disease. Prayer is generally practiced in conjunction with conventional medical care, but followers of some religions, such as the Christian Science Church, pray in lieu of using conventional medicine.

There has been a recent growth in interest about the possible medical relevance of prayer and spirituality. Some of this interest has been due to the research and writings of Dr. Herbert Benson and Dr. Larry Dossey. Important issues that have been raised are whether spirituality improves health and whether prayer can improve the course of a disease or lessen the severity of a specific symptom.

Treatment Method

Most religions involve some type of prayer. Praying may be done individually or in groups. It may be a type of meditation or may involve recitations of words silently or aloud. One type of prayer that has been studied in medical settings is known as *intercessory prayer*, which involves one person praying for another individual who may be in a different geographic location. It is important to recognize that prayer is one of many components of religious practice and that it may not be effective if done independently of the other aspects of religious belief.

In addition to prayer, spirituality is an active area of research. Whether spiritual belief produces effects beyond those of the placebo response has not been established. It has been claimed that spirituality may be an especially potent means of producing the placebo effect because placebo effects require belief and religious belief may be the most profound form of belief.

Studies of MS and Other Conditions

The effects of prayer and spirituality on MS have not been rigorously studied. One frequently described case of MS that appeared to respond dramatically to prayer and faith involved Rita Klaus. Klaus was a nun who was diagnosed with MS in 1960 at the age of 20. Because of the effects of her illness, she was given dispensation of her vows and left the convent. She eventually married and had three children.

Her disease progressed significantly over the years. She wore leg braces, required the use of a wheelchair, and eventually had surgery on her knees to relieve some of the severe stiffness, or spasticity, in her legs. Her religious faith dwindled with the progression of her disease. She became skeptical of God and religion in general.

At the urging of her husband, she became more committed religiously, prayed regularly, and developed a renewed and more mature faith. Then, one evening in 1986, 26 years after her diagnosis of MS, she prayed for healing of her disease. The following morning, she had unusual warm and itching sensations in her legs. She was able to move her legs and then get out of her wheelchair and walk. The surgical changes in her knees were no longer apparent.

Klaus has not had any recurrent symptoms of MS since that day in 1986. By this account, her MS became inactive, and she also recovered fully from the significant injury to her nervous system that had occurred over 26 years. She returned to her job as a schoolteacher and now gives public lectures on her remarkable experience. Her physician, Dr. Donald Meister, reported that her neurologic examination returned to normal. He is unable to explain her recovery. A urologist found that her urinary system, which had been very abnormal, had returned to normal function. The medical documentation of her recovery is reportedly under review by the Vatican.

A large, formal clinical study is under way in the Midwest to evaluate the area of prayer in MS more fully. This study of more than 200 people with MS is evaluating the effects of intercessory prayer on the disease course. There are two groups, one of which is receiving prayer while the other is not.

Variable results have been obtained in studies of the effects of prayer on other medical conditions. Anxiety and stress, which may occur with MS, appear to be reduced by prayer. This effect presumably is due to the fact that prayer, like meditation, elicits the relaxation response (see "Meditation").

One active area of investigation is the possible influence of intercessory prayer on people with recent heart attacks. Interest in this area was stimulated by a widely known study that was conducted in a coronary care unit in San Francisco (1). This 1988 study of nearly 400 people found that those who were prayed for experienced fewer complications, including heart failure, respiratory problems, and use of some types of medication. There was no effect of prayer on the death rate or the length of hospital stay. This study has been criticized for many reasons, including statistical flaws. A more rigorous study in a similar setting was reported in 1999 (2). In this study of 990 people in a coronary care unit in Kansas City, the people praying knew only the first name of patients, and patients were not aware of the study. As in the previous study, the prayer group had fewer complications but no change in the length of hospital stay. An even larger study of prayer in people with heart disease is currently under way in Boston. Under the direction of Dr. Herbert Benson, this study will involve approximately 1,200 people; the results are not yet available.

The effects of spirituality on MS have not been formally investigated. However, spirituality may be beneficial for anxiety and stress, which may occur with MS. Also, regular religious involvement has been associated with decreased depression in the elderly. On the other hand, other studies indicate that depression may be increased among those who are religious, especially Pentecostals, "non–mainline Protestants," and Catholics or Protestants who stop going to church. In a study of another chronic disease, diabetes, spirituality was associated with decreased levels of psychological distress and uncertainty.

Large surveys of studies of spirituality and health have been reported. One review of 115 studies of religious belief and health found that a positive effect occurred in 37, no effect occurred in 31, and a negative effect occurred in 47. A different analysis examined spiritual commitment and found that a positive health influence was associated with religious involvement in 22 of 27 studies. Some of the positive health effects of spiritual belief have been attributed to the social and community support that occurs with attending church. Many of the studies in this area have not been well designed. Further studies are needed to clarify the effects of spirituality on health.

Side Effects

Prayer and spirituality are generally safe. Some people have expressed concern that negative thoughts about an individual could lead to negative health outcomes. Prayer and spirituality should not be used in place of conventional medical care.

Conclusion

Prayer and spirituality are low risk and inexpensive. The health effects of these approaches have not been established. Some studies suggest that prayer may be beneficial for anxiety and that spirituality may be helpful for anxiety and depression. Research is currently under way to evaluate the effect of prayer on MS.

Additional Readings

Books

Benson H, *Timeless Healing: The Power and Biology of Belief.* New York: Simon & Schuster, 1996.

Cassileth BR. *The Alternative Medicine Handbook.* New York: W.W. Norton, 1998:292–293, 309–313.

Dossey L. *Reinventing Medicine: Beyond Mind-Body to a New Era of Healing.* San Francisco: HarperCollins, 1999.

Hirshberg C, Barasch MI. *Remarkable Recovery: What Extraordinary Healings Tell Us About Getting Well and Staying Well.* New York: Berkley, 1996.

Journal Articles

Easterbrook G. Science and God: A warming trend? *Science* 1997; 277:890–893.

Harris WS, Gowda M, Kolb J, et al. A randomized, controlled trial of the effects of remote, intercessory prayer on outcomes in patients admitted to the coronary care unit. *Arch Intern Med* 1999; 159:2273–2278.

Holden C. Subjecting belief to the scientific method. *Science* 1999; 284:1257–1259.

Roush W, Herbert Benson. Mind-body maverick pushes the envelope. *Science* 1997; 276:357–359.

Sloan RP, Bagiella E, Powell T. Religion, spirituality and medicine. *Lancet* 1999; 353:664–667.

$\mathcal{P}$rocarin

$\mathcal{T}$he preparation known as Procarin was developed by Elaine DeLack, a nurse with MS who lives in the state of Washington. It is claimed that Procarin improves many MS-related symptoms.

Treatment Method

Procarin contains histamine and caffeine and is administered by a skin patch applied to the thigh. A patch is used because histamine is not absorbed if it is taken by mouth. In one study, the patch was applied for eight hours, and two patches were used daily. In late 1999, it was estimated that 800 Americans with MS had tried Procarin.

Procarin was developed on the basis of a theory about histamine developed by Dr. Bayard Horton and Dr. Hinton Jonez in the 1940s and 1950s. Histamine treatment presumably decreases allergic reactions and enlarges blood vessels. Caffeine acts as a stimulant.

Studies in MS and Other Conditions

Information about the effectiveness of Procarin itself is limited. Elaine DeLack claims that her MS was dramatically improved by using Procarin. There are reports of a study of Procarin in 10 people with MS in Washington State. It is claimed that 8 of the 10 people in this study experienced improvement in MS symptoms that included bladder and bowel difficulties, incoordination, weakness, speech problems, walking unsteadiness, and fatigue.

One published study evaluated the effects of Procarin use in 55 people with MS (1). It was found that 67 percent of people experienced improvement in MS symptoms after six weeks of treatment. Improvement was noted in a wide range of symptoms, including weakness, numbness, walking difficulties, pain, fatigue, and depression. This study is limited by the fact that neither caffeine alone nor a placebo treatment was used. Also, the effectiveness of the therapy was determined by self-assessment, an approach that is subject to inaccuracy.

Older reports of histamine treatment for MS, published in the late 1940s and the early 1950s, used intravenous histamine along with another medication (tubocurarine), physical therapy, and allergy testing. Beneficial effects of this multimodality treatment were noted. However, the significance of these findings for histamine treatment alone is not clear because several different therapies were used simultaneously and strict clinical trial guidelines (such as the use of placebo-treated groups) were not followed.

In response to information about Procarin's reported benefits, the Clinical Advisory Committee of the Greater Washington Chapter of the National MS Society released a statement in 1999. In this statement, physicians and nurses expressed the opinion that they did not believe that Procarin was beneficial for their MS patients. They also had concerns that Procarin was being used *instead of* prescription medications with established effectiveness for treating MS.

Side Effects

Limited information is available on the safety of Procarin. The histamine in Procarin may potentially worsen asthma, and there have been reports that Procarin has caused severe asthmatic attacks. One person taking lioresal (Baclofen®) experienced irritability and loss of appetite while taking Procarin. Rashes have occurred at the site where the patch is applied. Procarin should not be used instead of conventional MS medications, especially disease-modifying medications such as Copaxone®, Avonex®, Betaseron®, and Rebif®.

Practical Information

Procarin is available only by prescription and costs $149 to $249 per month.

Conclusion

Procarin is expensive, and there is limited information about its safety and effectiveness. It should be avoided by people with asthma because it contains histamine.

Additional Readings

Journal Articles

Gillson G, Wright JV, Ballasiotes G. Transdermal histamine in multiple sclerosis. Part 1: Clinical experience. *Alt Med Rev* 1999; 4:424–428.

Horton BT, Wagener HP, Aita JA, et al. Treatment of multiple sclerosis by the intravenous administration of histamine. *JAMA* 1944; 124:800–801.

Jonez HD. Management of multiple sclerosis. *Postgrad Med* 1952; 2:415–422.

Reflexology

Reflexology is a therapy based on applying pressure to specific parts of the foot. It is similar to acupressure and shiatsu. In the United States, reflexology was initially developed in the early 1900s by Dr. William Fitzgerald, an ear, nose, and throat specialist in Connecticut. He named the treatment *zone therapy*. Subsequently, in the 1930s, Eunice Ingham, an American nurse and physical therapist, modified the method and named it *reflexology*. Her nephew, Dwight Byers, is one of the current authorities in this area and is president of the International Institute of Reflexology.

Treatment Method

Reflexology aims to diagnose and treat medical conditions. Specific parts of the foot are believed to correspond to different body parts. The application of pressure to reflex points (referred to as "cutaneo-organ reflex points") on the foot is claimed to affect specific parts of the body. The left foot is associated with the left half of the body, while the right foot is associated with the right half. There are no scientific studies to support reflexology concepts.

Reflexology is intended to improve health by increasing energy flow to specific parts of the body. In this way, it is similar to other healing systems that believe in a life force, such as traditional Chinese medicine and Ayurvedic medicine.

Reflexology is usually provided by a trained reflexologist. It also may be done individually. Sessions usually start with a foot massage and are followed by application of pressure to reflex points.

Studies in MS and Other Conditions

Clinical studies of reflexology are extremely limited. No formal studies have evaluated the effects of reflexology on people with MS, although there are anecdotal reports of people with MS benefiting from reflexology. Small studies of headache, impaired bladder function after surgery, and premenstrual syndrome have found positive effects, but these studies have serious limitations.

Side Effects

Reflexology is well tolerated, and there are no known serious side effects. It usually is not painful. However, one recent German study of reflexology in people after surgery found that the technique occasionally triggered abdominal pain.

Practical Information

Reflexology sessions are 30 to 60 minutes in length. There are several informational resources for reflexology. Books on the subject are available in bookstores and libraries. Information and lists of trained practitioners are available from The International Institute of Reflexology, St. Petersburg Florida, 813-343-4811.

Conclusion

Reflexology is a low-risk, low–moderate cost therapy. Since it has undergone little formal investigation for MS and other medical conditions, its effectiveness has not been established.

Additional Readings

Books

Cassileth BR. *The Alternative Medicine Handbook*. New York: W.W. Norton, 1998: 236–239.
Vickers A. *Massage and Aromatherapy: A Guide for Health Professionals*, London: Chapman & Hall, 1996.

Journal Articles

Oleson T, Flocco W. Randomized controlled study of premenstrual symptoms treated with ear, hand, and foot reflexology. *Obstet Gynecol* 1993; 82:906–911.

T'ai Chi

$\mathcal{T}$'ai chi, also known as t'ai chi ch'uan, was developed in China hundreds of years ago and is a component of traditional Chinese medicine. On the surface, t'ai chi appears to be simply slow body movements. In practice, it may provide some of the physical benefits of exercise and the relaxation effects of meditation. T'ai chi has been widely practiced in China for centuries and has recently become popular in the United States.

Treatment Method

T'ai chi may be done individually or in groups. A high level of strength and flexibility are not required because it is based largely on technique. T'ai chi consists of slow, rhythmic body movements. The arms are moved slowly and smoothly in circular movements while weight is shifted from one leg to the other and specific breathing techniques are used. A specified series of movements is known as a *form*. T'ai chi movements are claimed to balance the two opposite forces, yin and yang. Performing t'ai chi movements is believed to strengthen and balance the life force, known as "chi" or "qi."

Studies in MS and Other Conditions

A small 1999 study found that t'ai chi may be beneficial for people with MS (1). This study, conducted at the American College of Traditional Chinese Medicine in San Francisco, examined the effects of an eight-week t'ai chi group program on 19 people with MS. People were accepted into the study regardless of the severity of their disability. T'ai chi improved emotional and social function and produced physical benefits, with a 21 percent improvement in walking speed and a 28 percent decrease in muscle stiffness. Comments obtained from participants indicated that the group experience itself was an important component of the program. The results of

173

this study are promising, but there are limitations. Specifically, there was no placebo-treated group, and assessment was done by the participants themselves rather than by unbiased observers. Further studies are needed to investigate t'ai chi in MS.

The effects of t'ai chi on some MS-related symptoms have been investigated in other conditions. Most of the t'ai chi clinical trials have flaws and make it difficult to determine exactly how effective t'ai chi is relative to other forms of exercise. Most notably, t'ai chi has been found to be beneficial for improving walking steadiness in several studies in the elderly. In one study of 200 people, the risk of falls decreased by nearly 50 percent. Some of the effects of t'ai chi on walking may be due to increased confidence and decreased fear of falling. Research studies have found that t'ai chi also increases strength and flexibility. It may improve heart and lung function and decrease heart rate and blood pressure; it also may have a positive effect on mental function. There is limited evidence that t'ai chi improves depression, anxiety, fatigue, and confusion.

T'ai chi is an interesting example of a therapy that may be clinically effective in spite of the fact that its proposed mechanism of action—balancing and strengthening life energy—is unproven.

Side Effects

T'ai chi does not generally pose any known significant health risk. It could potentially worsen fatigue in people with MS. Also, walking unsteadiness and sensitivity to overheating may require modifications in technique. There is one report of a person with MS in whom t'ai chi provoked electrical sensations in the arms and back (known as Lhermitte's sign).

Practical Information

It is easiest to learn t'ai chi through classes. For people with significant disabilities, t'ai chi may be practiced, but the pace may need to be slowed. T'ai chi may be practiced individually after the basic techniques have been learned.

T'ai chi classes are often provided through community centers and health clubs and cost approximately $50 per month. Many books on this subject are available.

Conclusion

T'ai chi is a low-risk, low–moderate cost therapy. It may increase walking ability, decrease stiffness, and improve social and emotional functioning. Studies on other conditions indicate that t'ai chi increases strength and may improve fatigue, depression, and anxiety. For people with MS who have disabilities that prevent using strenuous exercise programs, t'ai chi may be a gentle way to obtain some of the general health benefits of a vigorous workout.

Additional Readings

Books

Cassileth BR. *The Alternative Medicine Handbook*. New York: W.W. Norton, 1998:243–247.
Fugh-Berman A. *Alternative Medicine: What Works*. Baltimore: Williams & Wilkins, 1997:197–199.

Journal Articles

Husted C, Pham L, Hekking A, et al. Improving quality of life for people with chronic conditions: The example of t'ai chi and multiple sclerosis. *Alt Ther* 1999; 5:70–74.
Wolf Steven L, Barnhart Huiman X, Kutner Nancy G, et al. Reducing frailty and falls in older persons: An investigation of t'ai chi and computerized balance training. *JAGS* 1996; 44:489–497.
Wolf SL, Barnhart HX, Ellison GL, et al. The effect of t'ai chi quan and computerized balance training on postural stability in older subjects. *Phys Ther* 1997; 77:371–384.
Wolf SL, Coagula C, XU T. Exploring the basis of t'ai chi chuan as a therapeutic exercise approach. *Arch Phys Med Rehabil* 1997; 78:886–892.

Therapeutic Touch

Therapeutic touch is an energy-based healing method in which life energy is believed to be manipulated therapeutically by the hands of a practitioner. Delores Krieger, currently an Emeritus Professor of Nursing at New York University, and Dora Kunz, a healer and clairvoyant, developed this technique in the 1970s. According to Krieger, therapeutic touch has been taught to more than 40,000 people and is practiced in more than 70 countries.

Therapeutic touch is based on concepts similar to those underlying the religious practice of "laying on of hands," in which healing energy is believed to pass from a healer to another person. Similarly, in therapeutic touch, a practitioner's hands are claimed to evaluate and beneficially alter an individual's "energy field." Therapeutic touch is based on a concept of a "life force," as are traditional Chinese medicine, Ayurvedic medicine, and some other healing methods. It is a modern variation of some of these ancient healing methods.

Treatment Method

Contrary to its name, therapeutic touch does not actually involve touching. Instead, the practitioners' hands are held two to four inches from a person's body. There are several components of the therapeutic touch session. After an initial "centering" procedure, in which a practitioner establishes an appropriate state of mind, the therapist's hands are used to evaluate the energy flow. Undesirable energy is subsequently removed by sweeping hand movements, and beneficial energy is transferred from the practitioner to the treated individuals. Sessions typically last 20 to 30 minutes.

Studies in MS and Other Conditions

There are many anecdotal reports of the benefits of therapeutic touch. However, there are very limited clinical studies of this technique. A few studies have been reported in major medical journals, and some studies have not found beneficial effects. The validity of therapeutic touch was recently questioned in a well-publicized article in the *Journal of the American Medical Association (JAMA)* (1). In this study, a 9-year-old girl, Emily Rosa, along with several other investigators (including her mother and father) evaluated 21 therapeutic touch practitioners. Overall, the practitioners, when blindfolded, were not able to detect when their hands were near the hands of another individual. This study, which has been criticized in several areas, questions the conceptual basis of therapeutic touch. A subsequent study of people untrained in therapeutic touch found that people could detect the location of an unseen hand if it was three or four inches away but not six inches away. Also, at three inches, a glass shield led to an inability to detect hand location. The authors concluded that body heat, as opposed to an "energy field," was probably used to determine hand location (2).

No large clinical studies of therapeutic touch have been conducted in MS. However, some symptoms that may occur with MS have been evaluated in small studies, reported primarily in nursing journals. Several studies of hospitalized patients found that therapeutic touch decreased anxiety, and small studies have reported improvement in depression. Mild beneficial effects in small studies have been reported for pain after surgery, tension headaches, burn-associated pain, and arthritis.

Therapeutic touch has undergone limited investigation in other conditions. Preliminary results indicate that wounds heal more rapidly in those who receive therapeutic touch. Therapeutic touch is endorsed as a comfort-promoting technique by the National League for Nursing. Some of its benefits may be due to the attention and caring of the practitioner. Clearly, more research is needed to determine the effects of therapeutic touch.

Side Effects

There are no significant adverse effects of therapeutic touch. Some practitioners believe that excessive energy may be transferred if a session is too long.

Practical Information

Practitioners of therapeutic touch may be found in the phone book under the listing of "Massage Therapists." More information about therapeutic touch and practitioners may be obtained from:

- Nurse Healers Professional Associates, Incorporated, 1211 Locust Street, Philadelphia Pennsylvania, 19107, 215-545-8079
- American Massage Therapy Association, 820 Davis Street, Suite 100, Evanston, Illinois 60201, 847-864-0123

Conclusion

Therapeutic touch is a low-risk, low–moderate expense technique. It has not been studied specifically in MS, and the effects of therapeutic touch on other conditions are largely unknown. Suggestive results of benefit have been reported for anxiety, depression, and pain, but further research is needed to determine the effectiveness of this therapy.

Additional Readings

Books

Fugh-Berman A. *Alternative Medicine: What Works.* Baltimpre: Williams & Wilkins, 1997:155–157.
Micozzi MS. *Fundamentals of Complementary and Alternative Medicine.* New York: Churchill Livingstone, 1996:121–136.

Journal Articles

Krieger D. Healing with therapeutic touch. *Alt Ther* 1998; 4:87–92.
Long R, Bernhardt P, Evans W. Perception of conventional sensory cues as an alternative to the postulated 'human energy field' of therapeutic touch. *Sci Rev Alt Med* 1999; 3:53–61.
Rosa L, Rosa E, Sarner L, et al. A close look at therapeutic touch. *JAMA* 1998; 279:1005–1010.

Toxins

Over the years, it has been proposed that many toxins may cause MS or worsen its symptoms. Recent reports have associated MS with aspartame use and mercury from dental amalgam, both of which are discussed elsewhere in this book. It has also been claimed that MS is provoked by cosmetics and by chemicals in the environment in the form of pollution, aerosol sprays, low levels of formaldehyde, and fumes from solvents. In food, it has been claimed that additives and low levels of residual fertilizers and pesticides may be important. On the basis of concerns about toxic causes for MS and other diseases, an entire field known as "clinical ecology" has emerged.

Treatment Method

Many approaches have been proposed to decrease exposure to specific toxins or to decrease levels of toxins in the body. Avoiding aspartame in the diet and removing dental amalgam are sometimes recommended for people with MS. Other approaches that are claimed to be beneficial for MS include detoxifying therapies such as chelation therapy and colon therapy, also discussed elsewhere in this book, and the avoidance of processed foods, tap water, aerosol sprays, potent housecleaning products, synthetic fabrics, and gas appliances.

Studies in MS and Other Conditions

There is no strong scientific or clinical evidence that a specific toxin plays an important role in causing MS or worsening its symptoms. The possible role of zinc or other metals in MS was raised by a study of workers at a manufacturing plant who were exposed to zinc and developed MS. Subsequent studies have not shown a definite association of MS with zinc or other metals. Similarly, there are no well-documented links between MS and aspartame or mercury (see sections on these topics).

When considering possible toxins and toxic injury to the body, it is important to recognize that the body has powerful tools to defend itself against toxins. The liver has biochemical mechanisms for converting toxic chemicals to nontoxic chemicals, and the kidneys are able to remove potential toxins from the body by excreting them in the urine. In addition, all cells in the body, including nerve cells, are very resilient and have mechanisms for combating toxins. Consequently, exposure to chemicals that can cause significant nervous system injury is believed to be extremely low, especially in developed countries.

Possible toxins in food have been investigated (1). Research studies have compared the cancer risk of pesticides in food with the cancer risk of chemicals that are naturally present in food. The natural chemicals in common foods, including peanut butter, mustard, and mushrooms, pose a cancer risk that is minimal but significantly higher than that resulting from the small amounts of pesticide in food. Also, the cancer risk of home air-conditioning is greater than that of pesticide in food.

Conclusion

No toxins have been identified that cause MS or provoke MS symptoms. Although a variety of techniques have been proposed to decrease toxin levels or to decrease exposure to toxins, there are no studies that demonstrate that these techniques produce clinical benefits for people with MS.

Additional Readings

Journal Articles

Ames BN, Magaw R, Gold LS. Ranking possible carcinogenic hazards. *Science* 1987; 236:271–280.
Schaumburg HH, Spencer PS. Recognizing neurotoxic disease. *Neurology* 1987; 37:276–278.

Tragerwork

Tragerwork is a form of bodywork. It is also known as Trager, the Trager approach, and Trager psychophysical integration. The technique was developed by Dr. Milton Trager, a physician as well as a boxer, acrobat, dancer, and follower of Maharishi Mahesh Yogi (see "Yoga"). Tragerwork is sometimes recommended specifically for people with MS and other neurologic disorders.

Treatment Method

Tragerwork is designed to change body habits that limit movement or produce muscle pain. With this treatment, an individual lies on a table while a therapist uses light massage in combination with shaking, bouncing, and rocking movements of the body. This process is believed to produce relaxation and allow one to move with less effort and more grace. Tragerwork therapists also provide instruction in "Mentastics" (a shortened version of "mental gymnastics"), a regimen of self-directed movements that maintain the feelings developed in the treatment sessions. Tragerwork attempts to increase freedom of movement through these methods.

Studies in MS and Other Conditions

Although Tragerwork is sometimes recommended for people with MS, it has not been specifically investigated in this area. There are anecdotal reports of benefit in people with MS, but few published studies have evaluated the effects of Tragerwork on any medical condition. One study found that people with lung disease had improvement in some measures of lung function after Tragerwork (1). The significance of this finding is not clear because the study was small and did not include a placebo-treated group.

Side Effects

Limited clinical studies have evaluated the effects of this therapy. Generally it appears to be well tolerated, but people with MS may experience dizziness and nausea with the rocking movements.

Practical Information

Sessions typically last 60 to 90 minutes and cost $65 to $90. A series of treatment sessions is often recommended. More information about Tragerwork may be obtained from The Trager Institute, 21 Locust Avenue, Mill Valley, California 94941, 415-388-2688.

Conclusion

Tragerwork is a low-risk, moderate-cost form of bodywork. Although there are anecdotal reports of beneficial effects from this therapy, it has not been formally studied in MS or any other medical condition.

Additional Readings

Journal Article

Juhan D. Multiple sclerosis: The Trager approach. *Trager Newsletter*. February 1993; 1–7.

Vitamins, Minerals, and Other Nonherbal Supplements

The use of vitamins, minerals, and other supplements is both popular and controversial. Surveys of people with MS indicate that the use of supplements is one of the most common forms of CAM. Much of their popularity probably is due to their accessibility. Supplements are easily purchased from grocery stores, health food stores, and drug stores, and using supplements does not require seeing a practitioner.

The potential benefits of supplements are frequently exaggerated by vendors and other proponents of supplements, and the possible uses of supplements in MS are sometimes based on incorrect information about the disease process. In conventional medicine, supplements have been viewed typically with skepticism. Supplements are now undergoing more serious investigation, and supplements are now recommended for preventing or treating a limited number of conditions on the basis of recent research studies.

Background Information

Vitamins are chemicals that are used for many of the body's fundamental chemical processes. In spite of the fact that they are present in only very small quantities, vitamins are absolutely necessary for normal body function. Thirteen vitamins are "essential," which means that the body does not have the biochemical machinery to synthesize them and that they must therefore be consumed in the diet. Most vitamins come from animal or plant foods. The 13 essential vitamins are the eight B vitamins and vitamins A, C, D, E, and K. Most vitamins are water-soluble. The four fat-soluble vitamins are A, D, E, and K.

Minerals are also important for maintaining the body's fundamental chemical processes. Minerals originate in soil and water and are incorporated into plants and animals. The minerals that are needed in large quantities, known as "major minerals," include calcium, chloride, magnesium, phosphorus, potassium, sodium, and sulfur. Those required in small quantities, the "trace elements," include chromium, fluoride, iron, selenium, and zinc. A total of 18 trace elements are considered essential.

In addition to vitamins and minerals, there are other types of supplements. Herbs are an especially popular supplement. Other categories of supplements include hormones, antioxidants, amino acids, and enzymes.

How Much Is Needed?

Much of the controversy in the supplement field centers around how much of a particular vitamin or mineral should be consumed daily. The Food and Nutrition Board of the National Academy of Sciences determines the Recommended Daily Allowances (RDAs), Adequate Intakes (AIs), or other similar values for vitamins and minerals (Table 1). These values, which have been revised recently, are the daily intake needed to prevent deficiency and possibly provide health benefits.

Some proponents of supplements claim that the RDAs are too low and that higher daily doses are needed. These higher doses of vitamins and minerals are known as "megadoses." In general, there is no strong evidence to support "megadoses." Importantly, high doses of some vitamins and minerals may produce adverse effects (Table 2).

TABLE 1. *Recommended Daily Allowance (RDA) or Adequate Intake (AI) for Adults*

Vitamins	RDA or AI	Minerals	RDA or AI
Vitamin A (beta-carotene)	4,000–5,000 IU	Calcium	1,000–1,200 mg
Vitamin B1 (thiamine)	1.1–1.2 mg	Iron	10–15 mg
Vitamin B2 (riboflavin)	1.1–1.3 mg	Magnesium	310–420 mg
Vitamin B3 (niacin)	14–16 mg	Selenium	55 mcg
Vitamin B6 (pyridoxine)	1.3–1.7 mg	Zinc	12–15 mg
Vitamin B12	2.4 mcg		
Vitamin C	75–90 mg, 35 mg more for smokers		
Vitamin D	200–600 IU		
Vitamin E	15 IU		
Folate	400 mcg		

IU, international units; mcg, micrograms; mg, milligrams

TABLE 2.   *Doses of Vitamins and Minerals to Avoid*

Vitamins and Minerals	Doses to Avoid
Vitamin A (beta-carotene)	Greater than 15,000 IU/day may produce multiple toxic effects; greater than 10,000 IU/day in pregnant women may produce birth defects
Vitamin B3 (niacin)	Greater than 35 mg/day may produce nausea, flushing, and other toxic effects
Vitamin B6 (pyridoxine)	Greater than 50 mg/day may produce nerve injury
Vitamin C	Greater than 1,000 mg/day may produce diarrhea and kidney stones
Vitamin D	Greater than 2,000 IU/day may produce liver injury and other toxic effects
Vitamin E	Greater than 1,000 IU/day may produce upset stomach and dizziness
Selenium	Greater than 200 mcg/day may produce multiple toxic effects

Are Adequate Amounts of Vitamins and Minerals Available in Food?

For a healthy adult, a well-balanced diet should be adequate because it contains enough vitamins and minerals to meet the RDA. It is not clear that supplements are necessary in this situation. However, supplementation may play an important role in other circumstances. For example, if the diet is not well balanced or is low in quantity, the RDA may not be met and supplementation is important. Also, people with certain conditions may benefit from vitamin or mineral doses that are higher than the RDA and may not consume these doses in spite of a well-balanced diet. Examples of this situation are folic acid supplements for pregnant women and vitamin D and vitamin B12 supplements for the elderly.

Vitamins and Minerals Interact with Each Other

There are several other significant features of vitamin and mineral supplements. First, there are complex interactions between vitamins and minerals. As a result, high doses of a single vitamin or mineral may be harmful or ineffective. For example, excessive vitamin C intake may affect the body's ability to absorb copper, and high doses of vitamin B1 may produce deficiencies of vitamins B2 and B6. Also, calcium cannot be utilized for bone health without adequate levels of vitamin D.

Supplements and MS

Supplements are one of the most popular forms of CAM used by people with MS. In addition to vitamins and minerals, a whole range of other specially formulated supplements is sometimes recommended for MS.

Several errors are frequently made in recommending supplements for use in MS. First, recommendations are sometimes haphazard and random; little or no justification is given for a long (and expensive!) list of supplements. When a justification is given, it is sometimes stated that MS is an immune disease and that immune-stimulating supplements are therefore needed. In fact, MS is an immune disease, but it is characterized by *too much*, not too little, immune activity. As a result, immune-stimulating supplements may actually be harmful for MS. Similarly, supplements that may affect the immune system are sometimes recommended for MS along with cancer and AIDS. Once again, all three diseases do involve the immune system, but people with cancer and AIDS may benefit from *stimulation* of the immune system, whereas people with MS may benefit from its *suppression*.

It is sometimes mistakenly assumed that if a deficiency of a vitamin or mineral impairs the function of the immune system or nervous system, an excess of that same vitamin or mineral will be beneficial to the immune system or nervous system and thus will be therapeutic for MS. In other words, it is assumed that if a little is good, a lot is better. In fact, there are probably very limited uses of high doses of vitamins and minerals.

A good example of this dosing issue that is relevant to the nervous system is that of vitamin B6 (pyridoxine). A deficiency of vitamin B6 impairs nervous system function. However, an excess of vitamin B6 *injures* the nervous system and may actually produce symptoms similar to those of MS. Thus, for vitamin B6 and the nervous system, a normal level is desirable, and either a deficiency or an excess may be harmful.

In the case of immune system function, seemingly paradoxical situations may arise with regard to supplement doses. For example, vitamin B7 (biotin) is important for maintaining a healthy immune system; a *deficiency* of vitamin B7 appears to be *beneficial* for animals with EAE, an experimental form of MS. On the other hand, supplementation with either selenium or zinc, two minerals involved in immune system function, may *worsen* EAE. On the basis of this limited scientific information, it could be argued that a state of deficiency of immune-relevant vitamins and minerals may be beneficial for MS, and a state of excess of these nutrients may be harmful. Because of limited information, it is not known if this argument is true. It is conceivable that it is true. Because MS is characterized by excessive immune system activity, deficiencies may be beneficial because they decrease immune system activity, and high levels may be harmful because they increase immune activity. This argument is not provided as a recommendation for people with MS to induce a deficiency state! Rather, it is provided to illustrate the complexities of vitamin and mineral dosing for specific diseases such as MS.

Vitamin and mineral supplements are clearly necessary for people with MS who have an inadequate diet. This may occur for a variety of reasons and may be particularly prevalent in those who are more severely impaired. With a poor diet, supplementation is essential to ensure an adequate intake of essential nutrients.

The most conservative approach to supplement use in MS is to avoid all supplements (except in people who clearly are nutritionally deficient). The rationale behind this view is that the effectiveness and safety of supplements has not been fully investigated in MS and therefore that supplements should not be used because they may be of no benefit and may actually be harmful.

Principles of Supplement Use in MS

Several steps should be taken when considering supplement use. Objective information should be obtained about the components of the supplement and the claimed health benefits. It must be recognized that in spite of some claims, no supplement has been fully investigated for benefiting MS. In addition, the use of supplements should be discussed with a physician.

Vitamins

Antioxidant Vitamins Generally (Vitamins A, C, and E)

Relevance to MS

Among all categories of vitamins, antioxidant vitamins were used most frequently by people with MS who were surveyed at the Rocky Mountain MS Center. Antioxidant vitamins include:

■   Vitamin A or beta-carotene (a chemical that is converted to vitamin A)

- Vitamin C
- Vitamin E

These vitamins act on *free radicals*, chemicals that can damage cells in the brain and other organs of the body. For years it has been proposed that free radicals may play an important role in aging, aging-related diseases, and many other conditions, including MS.

There is "good news" and "bad news" regarding antioxidant use in MS. The "good news" is that there is evidence that free radicals may be important in MS and that using antioxidants to decrease their harmful effects may be beneficial. In MS, one type of immune cell, the macrophage, injures the myelin coating on nerve cells by releasing free radicals. In addition, the axon—the central part of the nerve cell—is injured in MS, and free radicals may be important in causing axon injury. Also, immune cells are activated by the chemical products of free radical injury to the walls (or membranes) of cells. In an animal model of MS, EAE, there is evidence that free radicals are involved and that some antioxidant compounds decrease the severity of EAE. There is biochemical evidence of free radical damage in people with MS. Thus, there are multiple scientific and clinical studies indicating that antioxidants may be beneficial to the MS disease process.

The "bad news" about antioxidant vitamins in MS is that they affect the immune system in a way that may worsen the disease. In general, antioxidants stimulate the immune system, and the immune system is already too active in MS; MS therapies are designed to *decrease* the activity of the immune system. A variety of studies have shown that antioxidant vitamins, such as vitamins A, C, and E, stimulate components of the immune system, including cells known as macrophages and T cells. A similar stimulating effect has been observed with other antioxidant compounds, including pycnogenol, grape seed extract, and chemicals known as oligomeric proanthocyanidins (OPCs). The significance of this immune stimulation for an autoimmune disease such as MS has not been directly studied.

Limited research results are sometimes used as evidence for the safety of antioxidants in MS. One study found that antioxidant use (vitamin C, vitamin E, and selenium) for five weeks in 18 people with MS was *not* associated with worsening of the disease (1). However, this was only a single short-term study of a relatively small number of people. Another argument for antioxidant safety in MS is that EAE, an animal model of MS, appears to be improved with some types of antioxidant therapy.

Should people with MS take antioxidant vitamins? Some people argue "yes." However, given the possible stimulating effects of antioxidants on the immune system and the lack of studies of antioxidant safety in people with MS, it is not possible to give a definitive answer.

For people with MS, one reasonable approach is to *not* take antioxidant supplements and to obtain antioxidants through food, specifically fruits and vegetables. Current daily recommendations are two to four servings of fruits and three to five servings of vegetables. This dietary intake may result in adequate, but not excessive, levels of antioxidants and may provide other health benefits.

If people with MS choose to use antioxidant vitamin supplements, it is reasonable to take low doses. Low daily doses of these vitamins are:

- Vitamin A, 5,000 IU or less
- Vitamin C, 90 to 120 milligrams or less
- Vitamin E, 100 IU or less

High daily doses of certain antioxidants should definitely be avoided because of possible toxic side effects (see Table 2):

- Greater than 15,000 IU of vitamin A may produce multiple toxic effects, including headache, blurred vision, nausea, and liver injury.
- Greater than 10,000 IU of vitamin A in pregnant women may produce birth defects.
- Greater than 1,000 milligrams of vitamin C may cause diarrhea, abdominal bloating, and kidney stones.
- Greater than 1,000 IU of vitamin E may produce stomach upset, bleeding problems, and other difficulties.

There are other important precautions about antioxidant vitamin use. Vitamin A or beta-carotene supplements should be avoided or used cautiously by smokers because two studies indicate that beta-carotene supplements increase the risk of death and lung cancer in smokers. Vitamins C and E may inhibit blood clotting and thus should be avoided by people with bleeding disorders, people taking blood-thinning medications (such as warfarin or Coumadin™), and people undergoing surgery.

Because antioxidants are so popular and there are uncertainties about antioxidant effects on MS, a large-scale clinical study of people with MS is needed. Any result from such a study would have important practical applications. If antioxidant supplements are found to be beneficial, they could be recommended; if they are found to be harmful, their use could be discouraged; if they have no effect, they could be avoided and money could be saved or spent on some other type of treatment.

Vitamin E and Polyunsaturated Fatty Acids

It is sometimes recommended that people with MS increase their intake of polyunsaturated fatty acids, as discussed in the section on diet. Polyunsaturated fatty acid intake may be increased by modifying the diet or by taking fatty acid supplements such as evening primrose oil, sunflower oil, or safflower oil. A problem with polyunsaturated fatty acids is that they increase the need for vitamin E. As a result, if polyunsaturated fatty acids are a large part of the diet or fatty acid supplements are taken, supplementation with a relatively small amount of vitamin E may be necessary. It is recommended that 0.6 to 0.9 IU of vitamin E should be taken for every gram of polyunsaturated fatty acids consumed. Therefore, if one consumes 25 grams of polyunsaturated fatty acids daily, 15 to 22 IU of vitamin E are needed daily.

There is vitamin E in some polyunsaturated fatty acid preparations, including evening primrose oil. The label on the bottle of evening primrose oil should indicate the content of vitamin E.

Vitamin C

The Common Cold

It is sometimes claimed that vitamin C prevents or decreases the severity of the common cold. This is potentially important to people with MS because viral infections may trigger MS attacks. However, the effects of vitamin C on the common cold are unclear. Also, because vitamin C stimulates the immune system, high doses of vitamin C supplements are theoretically risky for people with MS. Because of its unclear effects on treating the common cold and its theoretical risks for worsening MS, it is reasonable for people with MS to be cautious about vitamin C use. If vitamin C is used, orange juice (50 milligrams of vitamin C per half cup of orange juice) or supplements in low doses (90 to 120 milligrams or less daily) may be reasonable.

Urinary Tract Infections

Vitamin C supplements are sometimes recommended for preventing or treating urinary tract infections (UTIs), which occur frequently in some women with MS. This recommendation is based on the idea that vitamin

C, also known as ascorbic acid, makes the urine acidic and thus inhospitable for bacteria. However, there is no definitive evidence that the use of vitamin C supplements produces acidic urine or decreases the chance of developing a UTI.

There is more evidence for cranberry juice (see "Herbs") than for vitamin C in preventing UTIs. If an actual infection is present, prescription antibiotics should definitely be used because people with MS may have serious complications from UTIs.

Vitamin D and Calcium

Vitamin D supplements may be underutilized by people with MS. Vitamin D has two important properties that are relevant to MS. First, it is involved in maintaining bone density, and people with MS are at risk for decreased bone density. Also, vitamin D acts to suppress the immune system and may thereby have a beneficial effect on the disease process.

Vitamin D is considered a hormone as well as a vitamin. A crucial step in the formation of vitamin D is sun exposure. In the skin, the energy of sunlight is used in a chemical reaction that produces the active form of vitamin D. Consequently, sunlight is necessary for adequate vitamin D production, and inadequate sunlight may lead to vitamin D deficiency. Only 10 to 15 minutes of casual sunlight exposure daily is needed.

Vitamin D is well recognized for its role in maintaining the health of bones. Vitamin D and calcium work together to make dense and strong bones. Low levels of vitamin D may lead to severely decreased bone density, a condition known as *osteoporosis*. A less severe form of decreased bone density is referred to as osteopenia.

Although many studies of osteoporosis focus on elderly women, it is increasingly recognized that osteoporosis affects many other sectors of the population. Among people with MS, there are several possible risk factors for osteoporosis and low vitamin D levels:

- People with MS are more likely to be women and to be less physically active than the general population; women and inactive people are at increased risk for osteoporosis.
- It has been reported that vitamin D intake is inadequate in 80 percent of people with MS and that blood levels of vitamin D are low in people with MS.
- Forty percent of people with MS may not have *any* sunlight exposure in an average week.

■   Steroids, which are sometimes used to treat MS attacks, may cause
      osteoporosis. The significance of this steroid effect is unclear in peo-
      ple with MS.

Given these multiple factors, one would expect an increased prevalence of osteoporosis in people with MS. In fact, this has been found in several studies. Bone density is decreased in people with MS, and the loss of
bone density over time is greater in people with MS than in the general
population. Based on bone density measurements, there is an estimated
two- to threefold increased risk of fractures in people with MS. There is an
increased risk of bone fractures with no known trauma in MS. These types
of fractures are indicators of decreased bone density.

Besides its effects on bone, vitamin D may have an important influence on the immune system. A possible association between MS and vitamin D deficiency has been proposed since the early 1970s. Because vitamin
D suppresses the immune system, it may be beneficial for MS and other
autoimmune diseases in which the immune system is excessively active. In
EAE, an animal model of MS, vitamin D supplementation prevents and
slows the progression of the disease, whereas vitamin D deficiency worsens
the disease. Interestingly, animal models of two other autoimmune diseases,
diabetes and lupus, are also improved by vitamin D supplementation.

There have been limited human studies of the effect of vitamin D on
MS. One older study evaluated the effect of vitamin D supplementation on
the frequency of attacks in 10 people with MS (2). Vitamin D treatment
decreased the rate of attacks. It is not possible to draw firm conclusions from
this study because it did not include a placebo-treated group and the treatment also involved cod-liver oil, which contains omega-three fatty acids that
may be beneficial for MS, as discussed in the section on diet. A more recent
preliminary study of 11 people with MS found that six months of treatment
with a form of vitamin D (19-nor) did not produce clear clinical benefits and
did not significantly decrease disease activity observed by MRI scanning (3).

Several geographic studies indicate a possible association of vitamin
D with MS. It is well known that the prevalence of MS generally increases
with an increased distance from the equator. Many hypotheses have been
proposed to explain this observation. One is that as the distance from the
equator increases, the sunlight exposure, and therefore the average level of
vitamin D, decreases.

Some studies indicate decreased MS prevalence with increased sunlight exposure. In Switzerland, MS is less common at high altitudes than at
low altitudes. There is more ultraviolet light exposure at high altitudes,
and perhaps this increases vitamin D levels and thereby decreases the risk

of MS. MS is relatively common in Norway except among people who live on the Atlantic coast. People on the coast are more likely to eat fish, which contain relatively high levels of vitamin D. It is possible that this dietary vitamin D protects the coastal people from developing MS.

If decreased bone density or decreased vitamin D intake is a concern, it should be discussed with a physician. Bone density may be measured by special diagnostic tests, one of which is known as bone densitometry.

Supplements of vitamin D are usually taken with calcium. The Adequate Intake (AI) of vitamin D is 200 to 600 IU daily and that of calcium is 1,000 to 1,200 milligrams daily. If vitamin D and calcium supplements are taken, the doses should be discussed with a physician or other healthcare provider. Prescription medications and, in postmenopausal women, hormone replacement therapy may be indicated. High doses of vitamin D should be avoided because they may cause fatigue, kidney damage, high blood pressure, and multiple other toxic effects. Also, calcium and iron should not be taken together because these minerals may interfere with each other's absorption.

Vitamin B12

For years it has been proposed that vitamin B12 deficiency plays a role in MS. Vitamin B12 is important for maintaining normal nerve function, and low levels of vitamin B12 may produce injury to the optic nerves and the spinal cord, two components of the nervous system that are also damaged in MS. However, this does not mean that vitamin B12 deficiency and MS are similar diseases.

It is sometimes assumed that people with neurologic diseases such as MS should take vitamin B12 supplements because vitamin B12 deficiency causes neurologic injury. This is not a logical argument. Low levels of vitamin B12 are harmful to nerves, but there is no evidence that high levels are any better for nerve function than normal levels. Of note, a small study of six people with progressive MS found that massive doses of vitamin B12 for six months did not produce any improvement in disability.

Studies of vitamin B12 levels in people with MS have produced variable results. It is clear from these studies that the majority of people with MS have normal vitamin B12 levels. There may be a small subgroup of people with MS who have low vitamin B12 levels. The cause for this low level in some people with MS is not known.

People with suspected MS should be evaluated for vitamin B12 deficiency because of the rare association of vitamin B12 deficiency and MS. Vitamin B12 levels should be evaluated through blood testing that is ordered by a physician or other healthcare provider. If the vitamin B12 level is normal, no further vitamin B12 testing is required and vitamin B12 supplements are not necessary. If the vitamin B12 level is low, further testing may be needed and vitamin B12 injections or pills may be indicated. The usual treatment for vitamin B12 deficiency is monthly injections of the vitamin. Oral treatment may also be possible. Lifetime therapy is often necessary, and follow-up vitamin B12 testing may be indicated on an intermittent basis.

Other B Vitamins

For unstated or illogical reasons, B vitamin supplementation is sometimes recommended for MS. The B vitamins include vitamin B1 (thiamine), vitamin B2 (riboflavin), vitamin B3 (niacin), vitamin B5 (pantothenic acid), vitamin B6 (pyridoxine), vitamin B7 (biotin), vitamin B12 (cobalamin), and folate (or folic acid).

B vitamins are sometimes recommended because they play an important role in the functioning of both the immune system and the nervous system. It is recognized that deficiencies of several of the B vitamins can produce serious disorders of the immune system and the nervous system. However, because a deficiency produces abnormalities, it should not then be assumed that an excess is better than normal levels.

Folic acid may play a role in regulating immune function. There are no consistent findings of decreased levels of folic acid in people with MS. In addition, there are no clinical studies demonstrating that supplements of folic acid are beneficial for MS. For people who take methotrexate, a chemotherapy agent occasionally used to treat MS, the toxic effects of the drug may be decreased by taking folic acid supplements.

At this time, there is no research evidence to demonstrate that people with MS in general benefit from B vitamin supplementation. As noted in the section on vitamin B12, a small subgroup of people with MS have vitamin B12 deficiency and should be treated. High doses of the other B vitamins should be avoided. In particular, excessive doses of vitamin B6 (pyridoxine) and vitamin B3 (niacin) should be avoided:

■ More than 50 milligrams daily of vitamin B6 (pyridoxine) may produce nerve injury. This may result in numbness and tingling in the hands and feet, which is similar to symptoms that may be experienced with MS. There is also a theoretical risk of immune stimulation with high doses of vitamin B6.

■ Greater than 35 milligrams of vitamin B3 (niacin) daily may produce flushing, nausea, liver injury, and increased blood sugar levels.

Multivitamins

Multivitamins are frequently taken by people with MS. Multivitamin preparations contain variable types and amounts of vitamins and minerals.

No rigorous clinical studies have examined the benefits or safety of multivitamin use in MS. Studies in elderly people indicate that multivitamin preparations may stimulate the immune system. This type of stimulation may theoretically be harmful for MS. However, the significance of this immune system effect for a disease process such as MS is not clear at this time.

A multivitamin preparation is important for people with MS who have an inadequate intake of vitamins and minerals. For people with MS with an adequate diet, the benefits of multivitamin preparations are not known. If multivitamins are taken, it is important to review the amount of each vitamin and mineral in a preparation. Obviously, toxic doses should be avoided (Table 2). Commercially available multivitamins do not generally contain toxic doses of any compounds, but some high-potency "designer" multivitamins may contain high doses of particular vitamins or minerals. For people with MS, it may be logical, although of no proven benefit, to use low doses of potentially immune-stimulating vitamins and minerals, including vitamin A, vitamin C, vitamin E, selenium, and zinc. Low daily doses of these vitamins and minerals are:

- Vitamin A, 5,000 IU or less
- Vitamin C, 90 to 120 milligrams or less
- Vitamin E, 100 IU or less
- Selenium, 20 to 50 micrograms or less
- Zinc, 10 to 15 milligrams or less

Minerals

Calcium

Calcium supplements are sometimes recommended for MS, often for unstated reasons. Calcium supplements should be taken by people with inadequate dietary intakes of calcium. Also, calcium and vitamin D supplements are indicated for people with MS who have osteoporosis or risk factors for osteoporosis (see "Vitamin D and Calcium" in this section). There are no other clear uses for calcium supplements in MS. It should be noted that calcium interferes with iron absorption; consequently, calcium and iron supplements should not be taken together.

Selenium

Selenium is a mineral that is sometimes recommended for MS. This recommendation may be based on its known antioxidant activity or on studies suggesting that people with MS have low selenium levels. It is not clear that selenium is a reasonable supplement for people with MS.

As noted in the section on antioxidant vitamins, antioxidant compounds may have several beneficial effects on MS. However, most antioxidant compounds, including selenium, activate the immune system, and this immune system stimulation may conceivably worsen MS. In fact, in one study of animals with EAE, an experimental form of MS, selenium supplementation *worsened* the disease course and *increased* the mortality rate. Also, the severity of the disease was the same for animals fed low-selenium and normal-selenium diets. The results of this study suggest that selenium supplementation may actually be harmful for people with MS.

The influence of selenium on MS itself is not known because no large study has ever directly examined the effects of selenium supplements on people with the disease. One small study found that treatment with selenium and several antioxidant vitamins did not produce adverse effects in people with MS. However, this study was too small (18 people) and too short in duration (five weeks) to be definitive.

Because of the limited information about selenium, it is not clear whether selenium supplementation is beneficial, harmful, or ineffective for MS. It may be most reasonable for people with MS to avoid selenium supplements until more information is available. Selenium may be obtained in the diet from seafood, meat, and whole grains. If supplements are taken, it may be best to take low doses, such as 20 to 50 micrograms or less daily. High doses (greater than 200 micrograms) should definitely be avoided because they may activate the immune system and may produce fatigue, nausea, dizziness, hair loss, tooth decay, and other problems.

Zinc

Zinc supplementation is sometimes recommended for MS. In fact, zinc phosphate was one of the earliest recommended therapies for MS. Zinc phosphate was used in the 1880s as a treatment by colleagues of Charcot, a French neurologist who played a major role in defining MS as a disease. At this time, there are no clear reasons for people with MS to take zinc supplements.

Some recent studies suggest that zinc lozenges may prevent or shorten the duration of the common cold. Other studies have not shown beneficial effects. With these mixed results, the effects of zinc on the common cold are not known. This possible effect of zinc is of potential importance to people with MS because the common cold and other viral infections may trigger MS attacks.

Zinc supplements are also sometimes recommended in MS because zinc is involved in the chemical pathway of polyunsaturated fatty acids, as discussed in the section on diet. This chemical pathway has been implicated in MS. However, it is not known if the pathway is indeed involved in MS, and it is not known whether zinc supplements are necessary for this pathway to function normally.

It is important to recognize that zinc may actually *stimulate* the immune system. This may be the mechanism by which zinc exerts its presumed effects on the common cold. Zinc activates several different immune cells, including macrophages and T cells. In fact, zinc supplements appear to increase the amount of brain inflammation in EAE, an animal model of MS. This suggests that supplements in humans may worsen MS.

A possible toxic role for zinc was suggested by a report of a relatively high occurrence of MS in a zinc-related industry in New York. Blood levels of zinc were increased in people in this facility. Studies of zinc levels in other MS populations have produced inconsistent results: Some studies show high levels, but other studies indicate low levels. A *deficiency* of zinc produced *benefits* in a mouse model of lupus, an autoimmune disorder like MS. This finding is consistent with immune stimulation by zinc.

Immune system activation by zinc could worsen MS. Given the fact that zinc has unclear benefits and that it may potentially stimulate the immune system, it is reasonable for people with MS to avoid zinc supplements or to use low doses of supplements—such as 10 to 15 milligrams or less daily.

Other Minerals

A whole variety of minerals are sometimes recommended for people with MS. Some studies indicate that people with MS have low levels of specific minerals, such as magnesium, zinc, and copper. The meaning of these results is not known. Before 1935, some recommended therapies for MS actually involved supplements of minerals, including antimony, arsenic, mercury, potassium bromide, potassium iodide, and thorium. At this time, no published clinical studies demonstrate a definite therapeutic effect in MS with supplements of these minerals or with supplements of other minerals, including chromium, cobalt, copper, iodine, magnesium, molybdenum, phosphorus, potassium (in various forms), and vanadium. Finally, gold or silver supplements have been recommended for MS. These are of no proven benefit, and silver supplements may actually produce serious toxic effects.

Other Supplements

5-HTP

5-HTP (5-hydroxytryptophan) is a type of chemical known as an amino acid. It is chemically similar to another amino acid, tryptophan. 5-HTP is sometimes recommended for depression as well as for many other conditions. Tryptophan itself was sold in the past, and contaminated batches produced a serious condition known as eosinophilia-myalgia syndrome. One study indicates that 5-HTP contains the same contaminant. It would be safest to avoid 5-HTP on the basis of this information.

Alpha-Lipoic Acid

Alpha-lipoic acid is an antioxidant compound. Like the antioxidant vitamins, alpha-lipoic acid acts to decrease the damage produced by free radicals. Alpha-lipoic acid is normally present in the *mitochondria*, the energy-producing parts of the body's cells.

Alpha-lipoic acid may have relevance to neurologic disorders. Unlike some chemicals, alpha-lipoic acid is able to enter brain tissue by crossing the barrier between the blood stream and the brain (blood–brain barrier). Some studies indicate that it may be helpful for a diabetes-associated form of nerve injury known as *polyneuropathy* and may be beneficial for other complications of diabetes. Studies of alpha-lipoic acid in other neurologic conditions are currently under way. There is limited information about the safety of alpha-lipoic acid, especially for long-term use.

No published studies have evaluated the effectiveness of alpha-lipoic acid in MS. As with other antioxidant compounds, alpha-lipoic acid may, in theory, be beneficial for MS, but it may also, in theory, activate the immune system and be harmful for MS. Also, alpha-lipoic acid is more expensive than antioxidant vitamins. If antioxidant compounds are taken by people with MS, the most economical approach is to take low doses of vitamins A, C, or E (see preceding).

Amino Acids

Amino acids are chemicals that are used to synthesize proteins in the body. Mixtures of specific amino acids known as *branched-chain amino acids* are sometimes recommended for MS. There is no evidence that people with MS are deficient in amino acids or that amino acid therapy is beneficial for MS. Inconsistent results have been obtained in studies of the effects of branched-chain amino acid use on mental and physical performance in athletes. Importantly, high doses (greater than 20 grams daily) may produce fatigue by increasing the amount of ammonia in the blood.

One specific amino acid, threonine, has been studied in people with MS who have muscle stiffness, or spasticity. Research suggests that threonine improves stiffness as measured by formal clinical testing. However, this effect is so mild that it is not noticeable to people taking the compound. Thus, threonine does not appear to be effective enough to consider its use for MS-associated spasticity.

Androstenedione

Androstenedione became well known to the public after the baseball player Mark McGwire acknowledged that he used it in 1998. Androstenedione is a hormone that is sold as a dietary supplement. In the body, it is converted to testosterone, the male sex hormone. Androstenedione is of potential interest to people with MS because it is claimed to increase strength and energy.

However, clinical studies do not support its claimed benefits. It is not clear that the doses used alter testosterone levels or increase muscle strength. Also, androstenedione decreases levels of HDL, the "good" form of cholesterol, and may thereby increase the risk of heart disease and stroke. Finally, some of the hormonal changes produced by androstenedione may increase the risks of pancreatic cancer in men and breast cancer in women. Many other possible side effects may occur with androstenedione.

Androstenedione should be avoided because of its unclear benefits and its multiple possible side effects.

Caffeine

Caffeine is of potential interest because MS may cause fatigue and caffeine may improve mental alertness. Caffeine is available in tablet form as a dietary supplement. The use of these tablets, coffee, and other caffeine-containing herbs is considered elsewhere in this book.

Calcium EAP

In the early 1960s, Dr. Hans Nieper, a German physician, developed a compound known as calcium EAP. It is also known as calcium-2-aminoethyl phosphate, calcium AEP, and calcium orotate. Thousands of people have apparently been treated with this compound. Most information about calcium EAP is available only from literature by Dr. Nieper (who died in 1998) or organizations affiliated with him.

Calcium EAP is one component of an approach to MS referred to as the "Nieper regimen." It is believed that calcium EAP allows necessary chemicals to interact with nerve cells and protects nerve cells from injury by the immune system and by toxins. Several other principles underlie the Nieper regimen, including claims that milk and several minerals (chlorine, chromium, fluoride, platinum) play an important role in MS.

The Nieper program recommends calcium EAP treatment along with other measures. Calcium EAP is initially given intravenously in a dosage of 500 milligrams per day for five days per week. It is then given long-term as a pill or as an every-other-day intravenous dose of 400 milligrams. Other recommendations include steroid treatment with prednisone (five to eight milligrams daily); vitamin and mineral supplements (some at high doses), including selenium and vitamins C, D, and E; avoidance of bright sunlight, alcohol, milk and milk products, evening primrose oil, aluminum, fluoride, and drinks that contain phosphoric acid or quinine; avoidance of water in the environment by not using waterbeds and hiring a dowser to be certain there is no underground water near one's bedroom; consumption of olive oil and raw food because of their "Kirlian positivity."

The first person was treated with calcium EAP in Europe in 1964; the first person was treated in the United States in 1972. No well-designed clinical trials of calcium EAP have been published. A document written by Dr. Nieper in 1968 describes the treatment of 167 people with MS. Beneficial effects were observed in 46 percent with mild disease, 33 percent with moderate disease, and 16 percent with severe disease. The overall benefit was 32 percent. Importantly, there was no placebo group in this study. Other literature by Dr. Nieper claims benefits in 85 to 90 percent of people with MS. Overall, there are no well-designed studies to indicate a beneficial effect of calcium EAP for people with MS.

The safety of calcium EAP has not been established. Of concern is a 1990 report in which a 53-year-old woman with MS had an abrupt cessation of heart and lung function (cardiopulmonary arrest) during intravenous administration of calcium EAP. She was resuscitated and subsequently developed serious kidney, liver, and bleeding complications.

By Dr. Nieper's account, 1 in 10 animals treated with calcium EAP develop kidney stones. Also, females gain weight and males became aggressive. Apparently, these side effects have not been observed in people. Some people treated with calcium EAP develop headaches and chills.

In conclusion, there is no rigorous published evidence that calcium EAP has beneficial effects. Calcium EAP may be very costly. There is one report of serious complications with intravenous use, and there are no studies documenting the safety of long-term use.

Coenzyme Q10

Coenzyme Q10 is also known as CoQ10 or ubiquinone. Like some vitamins, coenzyme Q10 is an antioxidant that may decrease free radical damage. Also, coenzyme Q10 may improve the function of mitochondria, the energy-producing components of the body's cells.

Coenzyme Q10 use has been claimed to produce many different health benefits. Some of these claims are not justified. Coenzyme Q10 may have applications to neurologic disorders. This compound is currently under investigation in a clinical trial of one degenerative neurologic condition, Huntington's disease. It may be studied in other neurodegenerative diseases in the future. Multiple studies indicate that coenzyme Q10 is beneficial for several heart problems, especially a condition known as congestive heart failure.

No large published studies have evaluated coenzyme Q10 in people with MS. As for the antioxidant vitamins (see earlier in this section), coenzyme Q10 may have beneficial effects on MS. However, like antioxidant vitamins, coenzyme Q10 stimulates T cells and macrophages, two types of immune cells, and may thereby adversely affect MS.

The effects on MS of antioxidant supplements such as coenzyme Q10 are not known. If antioxidants are taken, vitamins A, C, or E are more economical than coenzyme Q10. Coenzyme Q10 may decrease the effect of blood-thinning medication (warfarin or Coumadin™).

Creatine

Creatine is a supplement that is claimed to increase muscle strength and increase body mass. It is of interest because many people with MS experience weakness.

Creatine is made in the liver, kidneys, and pancreas. It is involved in generating energy for muscle cells and other cells in the body. Creatine is available as a dietary supplement and may be obtained in the diet by eating meat and fish.

There are limited clinical studies of creatine. In healthy people, creatine supplements may improve performance for brief, high-intensity exercises. There are no published studies of creatine use specifically in MS. In people with diseases of the muscles or peripheral nerves (nerves outside of the brain and spinal cord), limited short-term studies indicate that creatine may increase strength and decrease muscle fatigue.

Creatine is usually well tolerated, although there are rare reports of creatine-induced kidney failure. The safety of creatine use for longer than eight weeks has not been studied.

In summary, research indicates that creatine may increase muscle strength in people with diseases of the peripheral nerves or muscles. However, creatine use has not been studied specifically in MS, and the safety of long-term creatine use is not known. Thus, this supplement should be used cautiously by people with MS because its effectiveness and safety have not been established. A formal clinical study of the benefits and side effects of creatine in people with MS may be worth conducting.

DHEA

DHEA, or dehydroepiandrosterone, is a hormone that is available as a dietary supplement. It is marketed as an antiaging compound and as a "miracle cure" for many medical conditions. Claimed benefits of DHEA that are of potential interest to people with MS include improvement in fatigue, sex drive, and mood.

DHEA is a naturally occurring steroid hormone that is produced by the adrenal glands. DHEA may be important for aging because blood levels of DHEA decrease significantly as people get older. DHEA levels decrease by approximately 90 percent by the age of 85 to 90 years.

Studies on DHEA have not demonstrated definite benefits. For heart disease, DHEA may have a beneficial effect in men but a harmful effect in women. Some studies indicate that it may have an antidepressant effect.

There is limited information about the effects of DHEA on immune system–related diseases such as MS. No published studies have been reported with MS. However, another autoimmune disease, lupus, has been the subject of some studies. DHEA may be beneficial in a mouse model of lupus and may have therapeutic effects for people with lupus. Additional research in this area is necessary.

In spite of these possible effects on lupus, DHEA is of concern for people with MS because it may activate the immune system. It is known that immune system activity decreases as people age. Because DHEA levels also decrease as people age, it has been proposed that DHEA may have an important stimulating effect on the immune system and that the aging-associated decline of DHEA is the cause for the aging-associated decline in immune function. DHEA appears to attach to and stimulate a specific immune cell known as a T cell. These T cells are already too active in MS, so additional T cell stimulation with DHEA might be harmful.

DHEA has multiple possible adverse effects. It may increase the risk of developing heart disease or cancer in women. Liver injury is also possible. The safety of long-term DHEA use has not been studied.

There is no strong reason for people with MS to take DHEA supplements. No definite benefits are associated with its use. In addition, it carries a theoretical risk as a result of immune stimulation and may cause multiple adverse effects, especially for women.

Lecithin

Lecithin, or phosphatidylcholine, is a supplement that is sometimes recommended for MS. It is involved in several body processes and is a major component of cell membranes. Supplements of lecithin are made from soybean oil. At this time, there are no studies to indicate that lecithin therapy is beneficial to people with MS. Its safety has not been extensively studied. High doses (greater than 20 grams daily) may cause nausea, diarrhea, urinary incontinence, and a fishy odor.

Melatonin

Melatonin is a hormone produced in the *pineal gland,* a small gland in the brain. Melatonin is involved in regulating *circadian rhythms,* the regular daily cycles of the body such as sleeping and waking. Blood levels of melatonin are high at night and low during the day.

Many therapeutic benefits have been claimed for melatonin. Most studies have evaluated its effects on sleeping problems. For insomnia, some, but not all, clinical investigations have shown a therapeutic effect with melatonin. Studies of another sleep disorder, jet lag, have produced mixed results. No studies strongly support the use of melatonin treatment for cancer.

A possible role of melatonin in causing MS has been proposed. In one study, high blood levels of melatonin were associated with a later age of onset of the disease and a shorter duration of the disease. The significance of these findings in relation to melatonin causing MS or the effect of taking melatonin supplements on MS is not known

People with MS should be aware that melatonin may activate the immune system. The effects of melatonin on the immune system are not fully understood. However, specific immune cells called T cells have sites to which melatonin attaches, and some studies have shown that melatonin stimulates T cells. Melatonin has been proposed as a possible treatment for AIDS and cancer on the basis of its immune-stimulating effects. Also, melatonin treatment worsens a mouse model of another autoimmune disease, arthritis.

In summary, melatonin may be helpful for insomnia and jet lag. However, it has a theoretical risk for people with MS because it may stimulate the immune system. It would be reasonable for people with MS to avoid melatonin. If melatonin is used by people with MS, high doses and long-term use should probably be avoided.

Oligomeric Proanthocyanidins

Oligomeric proanthocyanidins, also known as OPCs, are antioxidant compounds. They are one of the main components in several antioxidant supplements, including pycnogenol and grape seed extract. As noted in the sections on these substances, it is not clear that the antioxidant effects of OPCs are beneficial to people with MS. Furthermore, they are more expensive than antioxidant vitamins.

SAMe (S-adenosylmethionine)

SAMe, or S-adenosylmethionine, also known as "Sammy," is a supplement claimed to be an effective treatment for multiple medical conditions. SAMe is a naturally occurring compound that is involved in fundamental biochemical reactions called "methylation reactions." These reactions also involve vitamin B12 and folic acid. SAMe has been commercially available for years in European countries, including Germany, Italy, and Spain. SAMe became available as a dietary supplement in the United States in the spring of 1999.

Multiple therapeutic effects have been attributed to SAMe. Multiple studies indicate that SAMe reduces depression, which is relevant because depression may occur with MS. However, the research evidence for SAMe as an antidepressant is not as extensive as that for another supplement, St. John's wort. The biochemical way in which SAMe may produce its antidepressant effect is not known.

It has been claimed that SAMe may be a treatment for MS. This claim is based on several observations of uncertain significance. First, a small subgroup of people with MS have vitamin B12 deficiency. Because SAMe and vitamin B12 are involved in similar chemical reactions, it is proposed that SAMe is beneficial for MS. In addition, SAMe is sometimes used to treat some rare genetic diseases that produce injury to the nerve cells in a manner somewhat similar to the nerve damage produced by MS. However, these arguments for SAMe treatment of MS are not well grounded. There is no evidence that abnormalities in vitamin B12 or SAMe play a major role in MS, and levels of SAMe are normal in the spinal fluid of people with MS.

SAMe is claimed to be a potential treatment for other neurologic disorders, including Parkinson's disease, Alzheimer's disease, and epilepsy. Current research does not support the use of SAMe for these conditions.

Other therapeutic effects have been attributed to SAMe. It has possible beneficial effects on liver disease and on pain and stiffness in people with osteoarthritis. Limited studies indicate that it may be helpful for *fibromyalgia*, a rheumatologic condition, and for a spinal cord disorder that occurs in people with AIDS.

In general, SAMe appears to be well tolerated. In clinical studies, no major toxicity has been reported in 22,000 people treated with SAMe. Minor side effects are nausea and anxiety. It has no known interactions with drugs or other supplements. Because the mechanism by which SAMe works is not clear, it is safest to avoid taking SAMe in combination with antidepressant medications.

Depression is a serious condition, and anyone who feels that he or she is depressed should be evaluated by a physician. Treatment with SAMe—or any other antidepressant compound—should be done in conjunction with a physician. In clinical studies of depression, the daily dose of SAMe has been 400 to 1600 milligrams.

Conclusion

People with MS should be cautious in their use of supplements. Among vitamins, vitamin D may be underutilized for osteoporosis. Antioxidant vitamins (vitamins A, C, and E) have both theoretical benefits and theoretical risks in MS. Vitamin C does not appear to be effective for the prevention or treatment of urinary tract infections. A small subgroup of people with MS may have vitamin B12 deficiency and should be treated with vitamin B12 supplements. It is reasonable for people with MS to avoid multivitamins with high doses of possibly immune-stimulating vitamins and minerals.

Among other supplements, SAMe may be effective as an antidepressant. Creatine may improve muscle strength, but its safety and effectiveness have not been established. Caffeine may conceivably improve MS fatigue, but this has not been formally studied. Calcium EAP is expensive and has no well-documented benefits for MS. Selenium, zinc, DHEA, and melatonin may activate the immune system and thus should be avoided or used in low doses. It is not clear that nonvitamin antioxidant supplements, such as alpha-lipoic acid, coenzyme Q10, and oligomeric proanthocyanidins, offer any benefit over less expensive antioxidant vitamins. Androstenedione may be harmful and has no clear benefits.

Additional Readings

Books

Cassileth BR. *The Alternative Medicine Handbook*. New York: W.W. Norton, 1998:60–78.
Dillard J, Ziporyn T. *Alternative Medicine for Dummies*. Foster City, CA: IDG Books, 1998:253–271.
Jellin JM, Batz F, Hitchens K. *Natural Medicines Comprehensive Database*. Therapeutic Research Faculty, 1999.
Sarubin A. *The Health Professional's Guide to Popular Dietary Supplements*. The American Dietetic Association, 1999.

Journal Articles

Abramowicz M (ed.). Vitamin supplements. *Med Lett* 1998; 40:75–77.
Grimble RF. Effect of antioxidative vitamins on immune function with clinical applications. *Int J Vit Nutr Res* 1997; 67:312–330.
Harbige LS. Nutrition and immunity with emphasis on infection and autoimmune disease. *Nutr Health* 1996; 10:285–312.
Mai J, Sorensen PS, Hansen JC. High dose antioxidant supplementation to MS patients. *Biol Trace Elem Res* 1990; 24:109–117.

$\mathcal{Y}$oga

$\mathcal{Y}$oga was developed thousands of years ago in India. It is related to the Hindu religion and was created as a spiritual practice. Yoga means "union" in Sanskrit and is believed to unite the mind, body, and spirit.

Treatment Method

There are many different forms of yoga. One of the more popular forms in the United States is *hatha yoga*. Three main components of yoga are breathing, movement, and posture. A series of body postures and movements, known as "asanas," are performed. Deep, slow breathing is done in conjunction with the body movements. Specific breathing exercises, referred to as "pranayama," are also done. Different types of yoga have different levels of exercise intensity and posture difficulty. In addition to these physical activities, yoga may include meditation, ethical guidelines, and diet recommendations.

In contrast to popular belief, the primary aim of yoga is not to attempt to assume difficult, contorted postures. People who are not able to maintain postures may still perform yoga. Postures in the standing or seated position are made easier by the use of "props" such as straps and wooden blocks. Yoga may be practiced by people who have *severe* arm and leg weakness. In this situation, emphasis is placed on head and shoulder movement, breathing exercises, and meditation. On the surface, this limited program may not appear to be yoga, but it does in fact focus on the same elements as more conventional yoga techniques.

Studies in MS and Other Conditions

Despite its popularity, there are only a limited number of research studies of yoga. Unfortunately, many of them are small or have significant flaws. The effects of yoga on symptoms observed in MS have undergone limited investigation. Anxiety and stress have been reduced in some studies; this yoga effect may be long-lasting. People with pain may benefit from yoga. There are reports of decreased muscle stiffness with yoga, but this has not been formally studied.

An active yoga program for people with MS in southern California has been developed by Eric Small and the southern California chapter of the National MS Society. Small, who has MS, studied yoga in India and England. He began practicing yoga shortly after he was diagnosed with the disease. His disease has been relatively mild over the course of 40 years. He has adapted classic yoga poses so that they can be done by people with significant physical disabilities. Many of the students in his program have needed walkers or wheelchairs. In interviews with people in his program, beneficial effects have been noted in both emotional and physical functioning. People have described improvement in depression, concentration, memory, sense of well-being, breathing, walking steadiness, strength, and stiffness.

Yoga has been investigated in other diseases. In asthma, yoga has been associated with decreased medication use, increased lung function, positive attitude, and relaxation. It may decrease joint pain and improve joint movements for people with arthritis. Yoga may be helpful for diabetes and may decrease heart rate and blood pressure.

Side Effects

Yoga is usually not associated with any significant adverse effects. However, yoga involving difficult postures or vigorous exercise should be done with caution by:

- Pregnant women
- People with fatigue, sensitivity to heat, or impaired balance
- People with significant lung, heart, and bone conditions

If meditation is considered, people with psychiatric disorders should discuss this therapy with their psychiatrist (see "Meditation"). As with all forms of CAM, yoga should not be used in place of conventional medicine, especially for MS disease management or significant MS-related symptoms.

Practical Information

Yoga may be performed in groups or individually. Yoga techniques may be learned in classes, which generally last 30 to 60 minutes. Group classes cost approximately $7, and private sessions are $25 to $35 per hour. Benefiting from yoga requires an ongoing commitment; several hours per week over weeks to months are generally required.

Yoga classes are often available through recreation centers, the YMCA, and schools. A listing of yoga teachers is available each year in the July/August issue of the *Yoga Journal* (2054 University Avenue, Berkeley, California 94704, 510-841-9200).

A video with yoga poses designed for people with MS is the *Pathways Exercise Video for People with Limited Mobility*. Information about the southern California yoga and MS program may be obtained from the southern California chapter of the National MS Society (310-479-4456). General information on yoga is available from several yoga organizations:

- The American Yoga Association, 513 South Orange Avenue, Sarasota, Florida 34236, 941-953-5859
- International Association of Yoga Therapists, 20 Sunnyside Avenue, Suite A-243, Mill Valley, California 94941, 415-332-2478

Conclusion

Yoga is relatively inexpensive and generally safe. Although it has not been rigorously investigated, it may improve anxiety, pain, and spasticity.

Additional Readings

Books

Cassileth BR. *The Alternative Medicine Handbook*. New York: W.W. Norton, 1998:248–251.
Dillard J, Ziporyn T. *Alternative Medicine for Dummies*. Foster City, CA: IDG Books, 1998:191–196.

Journal Articles

Despres L. Yoga and MS. *Yoga J* July/August 1997; 96–103.

Summary

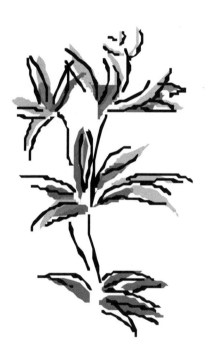

Integrating Conventional and Unconventional Medicine

There are many conventional medical therapies for MS and, as reviewed in this book, there are also a wide variety of possibly effective unconventional therapies. How can all of this information about different therapies be used to best advantage? One method is to consider each therapeutic area separately and to assess the relative merits of the conventional and unconventional approaches in each area.

The information in this chapter is not intended as a recommendation for CAM therapy. Any person with MS who is considering CAM therapy should always consider conventional medical therapy first and should thoroughly discuss any possible CAM therapies with his or her physician.

Precautions about CAM and MS should be kept in mind, as discussed in the introductory chapter. One precaution that is worth reiterating is that the information about nearly all forms of CAM is incomplete and that, as a result, pursuing CAM presents uncertainties and risks. Best guesses can be made about CAM therapies, but it is possible that some therapies that are now presumed to be "probably safe" or "possibly effective" will eventually be classified as "definitely unsafe" or "definitely ineffective."

Many different unconventional therapies are mentioned briefly in this chapter. More detailed information about these therapies is discussed in other chapters.

Disease Course

Therapies that can alter the course of MS are of widespread interest because they address the underlying disease process.

Conventional Therapy

Four immunologic therapies have been developed that alter disease activity: Copaxone®, Betaseron®, Avonex®, and Rebif® (not available in the United States). These medications have significant effects on the disease as assessed by clinical measures and MRI scans. All people with MS should be considered for treatment with these therapies.

Steroid treatment (by pill or by intravenous infusion) is typically used to attempt to decrease the duration of MS attacks and improve the ultimate outcome.

Possibly Effective CAM Therapies

CAM therapies in this area have not been as extensively studied as Copaxone®, Betaseron®, Avonex®, and Rebif®. Dietary approaches have produced promising, but not definitive, results. Therapies that are probably of low risk and of reasonable cost include:

- Diets—low saturated fat, high polyunsaturated fat, high fish intake
- Supplements—omega-3 fatty acids, omega-6 fatty acids

These therapies should not be substituted for conventional medical therapy. It should also be realized that the safety and effectiveness is not known for the combined use of these dietary approaches with Copaxone®, Betaseron®, Avonex®, or Rebif®.

Other CAM Therapies

Many other CAM therapies are sometimes recommended for improving the course of MS. Techniques that have not been well studied but are of low risk and low cost include prayer and spirituality, as discussed elsewhere in this book.

Two herbal therapies, Chinese herbal medicine and Padma 28, have produced promising results in small studies, but the effectiveness and safety of these approaches is unclear.

Ginkgo biloba is sometimes recommended for MS. Initial scientific and clinical studies of ginkgo biloba produced promising results for treating attacks of MS, but subsequently it was found to be ineffective.

Antioxidant compounds are sometimes promoted to improve the course of MS. Although these compounds may be beneficial, they may also be harmful because of their ability to stimulate the immune system. Antioxidants include:

- Vitamins—vitamin A (beta-carotene), vitamin C, and vitamin E

- Minerals—selenium
- Herbs—grape seed extract and pycnogenol
- Other supplements—alpha-lipoic acid, coenzyme Q10, and oligomeric proanthocyanidins

A variety of CAM therapies that are recommended for MS have not been studied carefully or are unlikely to alter the disease course but, at the same time, are reasonably safe. These therapies are aspartame-free diet, calcium, vitamin B12, and other B vitamins.

A long list of CAM therapies that have been suggested for MS are unstudied or are unlikely to be effective and also involve possible risk, high expense, or high levels of effort. As a result of these factors, caution should be used when considering these therapies. They include allergen-free diet and allergy desensitization, bee venom and other bee products, calcium EAP, Candida (yeast) therapy, chelation, colon therapy, craniosacral therapy, dental amalgam removal, enzyme therapy, hyperbaric oxygen, immune-stimulating supplements, melatonin, Neuralyn, Procarin, selenium, silver, spirulina, stinging nettle, toxin avoidance, and zinc.

Multiple (Five or More) Symptoms

People with MS may experience a variety of symptoms associated with the disease. These symptoms may be physical, such as muscle stiffness, weakness, or walking difficulties; emotional, such as depression or anxiety; or "invisible," such as fatigue.

Conventional Therapy

Conventional therapy is usually prescribed for one specific symptom. As a result, not many conventional MS therapies are effective for multiple symptoms. Physical therapy and occupational therapy may potentially improve function in a variety of areas, and some medications, such as antidepressant and anticonvulsant medications, may be effective for several different symptoms.

Possibly Effective CAM Therapies

In contrast to the symptom-specific or disease-specific approach of conventional medicine, CAM includes a number of therapies that are touted as being effective for many diseases or many symptoms. Although many of these multiple-symptom therapies do not live up to their claims, some CAM therapies for MS appear to be of low risk and have produced promising results for multiple symptoms:

- Acupuncture
- Biofeedback
- Cooling
- Exercise
- Hippotherapy
- Magnets and electromagnetic therapy
- Massage
- Music therapy
- T'ai chi

Other CAM Therapies

Some CAM therapies are claimed to be effective for multiple symptoms but have not been studied or are of uncertain effectiveness. Those that are of low risk include homeopathy, prayer, and spirituality. An aspartame-free diet is unlikely to be beneficial in this area but is also unlikely to be harmful.

Bee venom and other bee products are unstudied and may be harmful in rare instances. Multiple CAM therapies are unstudied or unlikely to be beneficial; at the same time they are possibly unsafe, expensive, or labor-intensive. Because of these concerns, these therapies should be fully investigated and well understood before using: calcium EAP, Candida (yeast) therapy, chelation therapy, dental amalgam removal, DHEA, hyperbaric oxygen, Procarin, and toxin avoidance.

Anxiety and Stress

Anxiety and stress may occur in association with MS.

Conventional Medical Therapy

Conventional medical therapy in this area is often very effective. It typically involves the use of anti-anxiety medications and possibly psychotherapy.

Possibly Effective CAM Therapies

Anxiety and stress may be due to multiple causes, some of which may be the result of medical conditions. As a result, a physician should be consulted about the possible causes before considering CAM therapies.

In general, CAM therapies for anxiety have not been studied extensively. The evidence supporting the use of conventional medical therapy, especially antianxiety medications, is much stronger than that for CAM therapy. CAM therapies that have yielded promising results are:

- Acupuncture
- Aromatherapy
- Ayurveda
- Biofeedback
- Exercise
- Feldenkrais
- Guided imagery
- Hypnosis
- Kava kava
- Massage
- Meditation
- Music therapy
- Prayer
- Spirituality
- T'ai chi
- Therapeutic touch
- Yoga

Other CAM Therapies

Homeopathy is generally safe but is of uncertain effectiveness for anxiety. Valerian is sometimes recommended for anxiety, but most studies of this herb have been for insomnia.

Bladder Problems

MS may affect bladder function in several ways, including problems with storing urine, emptying urine, incontinence, and urinary tract infections.

Conventional Therapy

Conventional therapy for these difficulties usually involves medications and lifestyle changes. Catheterization and surgical therapies may be indicated for more severe difficulties.

Possibly Effective CAM Therapies

People with recurrent urinary tract infections should undergo a medical evaluation because it is important to determine the underlying cause. A CAM approach may be reasonable in some situations and should be discussed with a physician. Cranberry juice may be effective for preventing urinary tract infections and is of low risk. Its effectiveness relative to the conventional approach with prescription antibiotics has not been investigated.

Conventional treatment with antibiotics should be used to treat urinary tract infections. One reason for this is that the effectiveness of CAM approaches for treating infections, including cranberry juice, is not established. Also, people with MS with urinary tract infections should attempt to eliminate the infection as quickly as possible because the infection may worsen neurologic symptoms.

It is important to undergo a medical evaluation for urinary incontinence. Because CAM therapies have not been extensively studied, it is important to consider conventional therapy first in this area. Multiple CAM therapies have produced promising results for urinary incontinence:

- Acupuncture
- Biofeedback
- Cooling
- Exercise (Kegel exercises)
- Hippotherapy
- Magnets and electromagnetic therapy

Other CAM Therapies

Vitamin C is sometimes recommended for preventing and treating urinary tract infections. However, studies do not indicate that vitamin C is effective, and it carries a theoretical risk in MS because of its immune-stimulating activity. Bearberry, or uva ursi, is also sometimes recommended for urinary tract infections. The effectiveness and safety of this herb have not been established.

Bowel Problems

There are several MS-associated bowel problems, the most common of which is constipation. Rarely, diarrhea or incontinence may occur.

Conventional Therapy

The conventional therapy of bowel problems usually involves developing a "bowel program," with changes in food and fluid intake and possibly treatment with medications.

Possibly Effective CAM Therapies

Low-risk therapies for constipation are psyllium seed and other herbs. A conventional medical evaluation is important for incontinence of stool.

Simple conventional measures are often quite effective. If CAM therapy is considered, those that have produced promising results in limited studies are:

- Biofeedback
- Exercise
- Hippotherapy

Colds and Flu—Prevention or Decreasing Duration

Colds and flu are of interest to people with MS because these viral infections may be associated with attacks. Any measure that prevents or decreases the duration of colds and flu may be helpful.

Conventional Therapy

Conventional medical approaches in this area include flu vaccination and recently developed flu medications (Relenza® and Tamiflu®). Also, infection with cold or flu viruses may be prevented by simple measures such as avoiding exposure to infected people, frequent hand washing, and avoiding touching the face with the hands.

CAM Therapies

Despite some claims, there is no magic CAM cure for colds and flu. No CAM therapy for the flu has been shown to be as effective as the medications that are currently available. As a result, people with MS who have flu symptoms should first consider these medications before CAM therapy.

Homeopathy is low risk but of unproven benefit in this area. A variety of supplements have produced positive results in some, but not all, studies. However, these therapies are theoretically risky for people with MS because they may stimulate the immune system and thus may potentially worsen MS. These therapies are echinacea, garlic, vitamin C, and zinc.

Coordination Problems

In MS, coordination may be impaired in the arms and legs. Several factors may contribute to incoordination, including tremor, weakness, muscle stiffness, and numbness.

Conventional Therapy

Mainstream approaches to incoordination usually involve occupational therapy measures, such as the use of special devices and compensatory techniques.

Possibly Effective CAM Therapies

Small studies in people with MS and in people with other conditions suggest that some CAM therapies may improve or compensate for incoordination. These include:

- Cooling
- Music therapy
- Pets

Other CAM Therapies

One low-risk CAM therapy that is claimed to be effective in this area but that has not been well studied is Feldenkrais.

Depression

Many people with MS experience depression. This condition may be serious and, consequently, should be evaluated and treated by a physician.

Conventional Therapy

Conventional therapy for depression is definitely effective and includes antidepressant medication and psychotherapy.

Possibly Effective CAM Therapies

As mentioned, complaints of depression warrant evaluation by a conventional medical approach. For mild to moderate depression, some CAM therapies may be considered with the supervision of a physician. Two low-risk and low-cost therapies that are probably effective are:

- Exercise
- St. John's wort

Many other CAM therapies are possibly effective and of low risk. Further studies are needed to determine whether these therapies are truly effective. They include:

- Acupuncture
- Aromatherapy
- Ayurveda
- Hippotherapy
- Massage
- Meditation
- Music therapy
- SAMe
- Spirituality
- T'ai chi
- Therapeutic touch

Other CAM Therapies

Homeopathy is safe but of uncertain effectiveness for depression. One dietary supplement, 5-HTP, is possibly beneficial but also may be unsafe. DHEA is of unproven benefit and may be harmful.

Fatigue

MS-associated fatigue is common and may be quite disabling. There are multiple causes for fatigue, including the MS disease process itself, depression, medication effects, and other medical conditions.

Conventional Therapy

Because of the multiple factors involved in fatigue, a physician or other healthcare provider should assess this symptom and determine the best treatment options. Mainstream therapy for fatigue, which is often quite effective, includes lifestyle modifications and medications.

Possibly Effective CAM Therapies

After a medical evaluation, CAM therapy may be considered for mild fatigue or for fatigue that does not respond to conventional treatment. There are several possible CAM therapy options, none of which have undergone rigorous evaluation in MS:

- Caffeine-including caffeine tablets, coffee, and other caffeine-containing herbs
- Cooling
- Exercise

■   Magnets and electromagnetic therapy
■   T'ai chi

Other CAM Therapies

Homeopathy is a low-risk therapy for fatigue that is of uncertain effectiveness. Asian ginseng may be effective for fatigue but may also activate the immune system.

Several supplements are of uncertain benefit for fatigue and may be unsafe. These include androstenedione, DHEA, Siberian ginseng, and spirulina.

Osteoporosis

As a result of inactivity, steroid use, limited sun exposure, and other factors, people with MS may be at risk for developing osteoporosis, a decrease in the density of bone tissue. A milder form of this same bone condition, osteopenia, may also occur.

Conventional Therapies

Mainstream therapy involves a variety of prescription medications along with calcium and vitamin D. In postmenopausal women, hormone replacement therapy is also considered.

Possibly Effective CAM Therapies

During conventional medical visits, osteoporosis is not always strongly considered in people with MS. Also, the use of vitamin D and calcium may not be seriously considered for people with osteopenia (a mild form of bone tissue loss) or for those with normal bone tissue and risk factors for osteoporosis. For these reasons, recognition and treatment or prevention of osteoporosis may conceivably be considered "alternative." Simple approaches that are effective, inexpensive, and safe are:

■   Exercise
■   Vitamin D and calcium

Pain—General

Pain is relatively common with MS. It may be caused by MS lesions in the nervous system or by weakness or stiffness that produce pain in the joints or muscles.

Conventional Therapy

The mainstream treatment of pain depends on its type and severity. Therapies include anti-inflammatory medications, specific medications that are effective for nerve-related pain, and physical therapy.

Possibly Effective CAM Therapies

CAM approaches may be worth considering if pain is mild or not completely alleviated by conventional approaches. Low-risk therapies that have produced promising results are:

- Acupuncture
- Ayurveda
- Biofeedback
- Guided imagery
- Hypnosis
- Magnets and electromagnetic therapy
- Massage
- Meditation
- Music therapy
- Therapeutic touch
- Yoga

Other CAM Therapies

Feldenkrais and homeopathy are generally safe but are of uncertain effectiveness for MS-related pain.

Pain—Low Back

People with MS may develop low back pain. This frequently is caused by strain of low back muscles as a result of weakness or stiffness in the legs. A more serious cause of low back pain is a herniated disk.

Conventional Therapy

In conventional medicine, low back pain is usually managed with physical therapy, anti-inflammatory medications, and muscle-relaxing medications.

Possibly Effective CAM Therapies

Because of the multiple possible causes of low back pain, a general medical evaluation should be done before considering CAM. This evaluation will determine if there is a serious condition, such as a herniated disk.

Some CAM therapies may be reasonable to consider for mild, uncomplicated low back pain or for low back pain that is refractory to treatment with conventional therapies. Two therapies that appear to be effective and are of low risk are:

■   Acupuncture
■   Chiropractic therapy

Two other low-risk therapies may also be beneficial for low back pain:

■   Exercise
■   Massage

Sexual Problems

MS may cause sexual difficulties, including decreased libido, erection difficulties, and reduced genital sensation. There may also be physical or psychological causes for these sexual problems.

Conventional Therapy

Because of the complexities in this area, conventional medical evaluation attempts first to identify the underlying problem and then to provide appropriate treatment. Conventional measures include medications, lubricants, sexual techniques, and counseling.

Possibly Effective CAM Therapies

Because sexual difficulties in MS are complicated, it is best to be evaluated by a physician or other healthcare provider. Few CAM therapies have been examined in this area. Cooling has produced suggestive results, but further studies are needed to determine whether it is definitely effective.

Other CAM Therapies

Yohimbe, an herbal supplement, may be beneficial for erectile difficulties, but it may also produce significant side effects. DHEA, another supplement, is claimed to be helpful for sexual difficulties. It is of unclear benefit, however, and may lead to adverse effects.

Sleep Problems

Sleep problems are more likely to occur in people with MS than in the general population. Stiffness and spasms may contribute to sleeping difficulties, and lack of sleep may cause fatigue. Many other factors are also related to sleep difficulties in people with MS.

Conventional Therapy

A conventional medical evaluation for a sleep problem initially involves determining its underlying cause. Treatment includes medications that promote sleep and medications and other measures that improve symptoms that may interfere with sleep, such as spasms.

Possibly Effective CAM Therapies

A mainstream medical evaluation should be obtained for sleeping problems. CAM therapies may be considered for mild sleeping difficulties or those that are not fully responsive to mainstream measures. Low-risk treatments with possible effectiveness in this area are:

■ Biofeedback
■ Exercise
■ Meditation
■ Valerian

Other CAM Therapies

Homeopathy is a low-risk approach that is of uncertain effectiveness for sleep problems. Several supplements are promoted for insomnia. As discussed elsewhere in this book, melatonin may be beneficial, but in people with MS it is associated with a theoretical risk because of its immune-stimulating activity. 5-HTP, another supplement, has unclear effectiveness for insomnia and may be harmful. Kava kava is sometimes recommended for insomnia, but most studies of this herb have actually only evaluated its effectiveness for anxiety.

Spasticity (Muscle Stiffness)

MS may cause spasticity, or muscle stiffness. This usually is due to MS-associated nervous system injury. MS may also produce spasms, a related symptom that is characterized by brief, strong muscle contractions.

Conventional Therapy

The mainstream approach to spasticity frequently begins with simple exercise techniques developed by a physical therapist. Medications such as lioresal (Baclofen®) and tizanidine (Zanaflex®) are often used. Injections of medications or other specialized therapeutic techniques are used for severe spasticity that does not respond to treatment with medications.

Possibly Effective CAM Therapies

No CAM therapies have been studied extensively for spasticity. It is unlikely that any form of CAM will relieve moderate or severe spasticity; conventional therapy should definitely be used. CAM therapy may be worth considering for spasticity that cannot be fully managed with conventional therapy or for mild spasticity. Low-risk therapies that have produced promising results in small studies include:

- Ayurveda
- Biofeedback
- Cooling
- Exercise
- Hippotherapy
- Magnets and electromagnetic therapy
- Massage
- T'ai chi
- Yoga

Other CAM Therapies

Pilates is a low-risk therapy that is claimed to be effective in this area but has not been formally studied. Marijuana has produced positive results in small studies. However, it may also produce adverse effects, and it is illegal in most states.

Thinking (Cognitive) Problems

MS may affect the brain in such a way that thinking difficulties develop. MS may impair memory and the ability to perform multiple tasks.

Conventional Therapy

A conventional approach to cognitive problems includes evaluation of cognitive function and assessment for depression or anxiety, both of which may affect thinking processes. Treatment may involve rehabilitation in identified areas of weakness and appropriate therapy for significant depression or anxiety. No prescription medications that definitely improve MS-associated cognitive difficulties are available.

Possibly Effective CAM Therapies

Limited studies in people with MS have indicated beneficial effects with:

- Cooling
- Magnets and electromagnetic therapy

Both of these therapies pose little risk. Further studies are needed to evaluate whether they are definitely effective.

Other CAM Therapies

Two other CAM therapies, ginkgo biloba and music therapy, are associated with minimal risks and have produced beneficial cognitive effects in other groups of people, especially the elderly. These therapies have not been specifically studied in MS.

Walking Problems

MS often causes walking difficulties. This may be the result of impaired leg function caused by weakness, stiffness, clumsiness, or numbness.

Conventional Therapy

The evaluation and treatment of walking difficulties is generally done by physical therapists. Treatment usually involves an individualized physical therapy program. Other measures include medications for spasticity and assistive devices such as braces, canes, and walkers.

Possibly Effective CAM Therapies

It may be reasonable to consider CAM for walking difficulties that are mild or do not respond well to mainstream approaches. In limited studies, multiple low-risk CAM therapies have produced promising beneficial effects for people with walking difficulties:

- Cooling
- Exercise

- Hippotherapy
- Magnets and electromagnetic therapy
- Music therapy
- Pets
- T'ai Chi

Other CAM Therapies

Feldenkrais is a low-risk therapy that is claimed to be effective for walking difficulties but has not been well studied.

Weakness

The nervous system injury in MS frequently produces weakness of the arms and legs. A lack of physical activity may also produce weakness through a process of physical deconditioning.

Conventional Therapy

Conventional medicine relies on physical therapists to determine which muscles are weak and to develop an individualized exercise program to strengthen these muscles.

Possibly Effective CAM Therapies

CAM therapies should not be relied on for severe weakness. It may be reasonable to use CAM for mild weakness or for weakness that does not respond significantly to conventional therapy. Limited studies in MS and other conditions indicate that several therapies may improve or compensate for weakness:

- Acupuncture
- Cooling
- Exercise
- Hippotherapy
- Pets
- T'ai chi

Other CAM Therapies

Creatine and the Pilates method are two low-risk CAM therapies that theoretically might be effective for weakness but are relatively unstudied. Androstenedione, a supplement that has been claimed to increase strength, has not been shown to be effective and may actually be harmful.

Conclusion

A Wellness Approach

It is important not to rely too heavily on CAM therapy for MS. There are other treatment options. Conventional therapy has many effective approaches for treating both the disease process itself and its symptoms. In addition, a more inclusive "wellness approach," which may include CAM, may also be taken. Although there are a variety of definitions of wellness, a wellness approach of value in MS is one that uses many different conventional and unconventional methods to optimize functioning in the different areas of one's life.

Health is one of these components; other important components include physical fitness, psychological well-being, social "connectedness," nutrition, sexuality, spirituality, and bowel and bladder function. These components are interwoven, and in a state of wellness there is a sense of wholeness and balance between them. A chronic disease such as MS may disrupt this wholeness and balance. Medical care can improve the health component, while a wellness approach may produce benefits in the other areas. Assessing these other areas and providing therapy requires a multidisciplinary approach and an openness to a variety of treatment techniques. This combined approach often requires medical, psychological, nursing, dietetic, and rehabilitation services.

Craze or Cure?

Is CAM use for MS a craze or a cure? The answer is "neither." Each specific therapy needs to be evaluated with respect to MS. Some therapies may be beneficial, others are ineffective or unsafe, and a large number have yet to be studied carefully in people with MS. This large variability and the possible effectiveness of different therapies is the cause for much of the confusion and controversy in CAM. Improving how CAM is used involves increasing communication between patients and healthcare professionals, developing accurate MS-relevant CAM information, and conducting reliable studies to determine the effectiveness and safety of CAM therapies.

Additional Readings

Books

Benson H, Stuart E. *The Wellness Book: The Comprehensive Guide to Maintaining Health and Treating Stress-Related Illness.* New York: Simon & Schuster, 1992.
Kraft, GH, Catanzaro M. *Living with Multiple Sclerosis: A Wellness Approach.* 2nd ed. New York: Demos, 2000.

Summary of the Effects
of Popular Supplements*

Alfalfa: immune-stimulating

Aloe: may interact with steroids

Alpha-lipoic acid: possibly immune-stimulating

Androstenedione: multiple possible toxic effects

Asian ginseng: no definite therapeutic effects; immune-stimulating; possibly fatigue-producing; may interact with steroids; may inhibit blood clotting; may interact with warfarin (Coumadin™)

Astragalus: immune-stimulating

Bayberry: may interact with steroids

Bearberry: also known as uva ursi; possible liver toxicity

Bee pollen: no definite therapeutic effects; rarely causes severe allergic reactions

Beta-carotene: see Vitamin A

Bissy nut: see Cola nut

Black currant seed oil: contains gamma-linolenic acid; unknown safety

Blue-green algae: see Spirulina

Borage seed oil: possibly immune-suppressing; contains gamma-linolenic acid; possible liver toxicity; may cause seizures

Caffeine: improves mental alertness; may irritate urinary tract

Cat's claw: immune-stimulating

---

*This summary provides limited information about popular supplements. See the index for a more complete listing of popular and nonpopular supplements covered in this book. See the text itself for more detailed information on supplements.

231

Chamomile: possibly fatigue-producing

Chaparral: possible liver toxicity

Cod-liver oil: possibly immune-suppressing; contains omega-three fatty acids; may inhibit blood clotting; may interact with warfarin (Coumadin™)

Coenzyme Q10: immune-stimulating; may interact with warfarin (Coumadin™)

Coffee: contains caffeine; improves mental alertness; may irritate urinary tract

Cola nut: also known as bissy nut; contains caffeine; improves mental alertness; may irritate urinary tract

Comfrey: possible liver toxicity

Cranberry: possibly effective to *prevent* urinary tract infections; should not be used to treat urinary tract infections

Creatine: possibly effective for weakness; unstudied in MS; unknown safety

DHEA: also known as dehydroepiandrosterone; possibly immune-stimulating

Echinacea: not definitely effective for treating viral infections; immune-stimulating; possible liver toxicity when taken with methotrexate

Ephedra: see Ma huang

Evening primrose oil: possibly immune-suppressing; contains gamma-linolenic acid; may cause seizures; may inhibit blood clotting; may interact with warfarin (Coumadin™)

Fish oil: possibly immune-suppressing; contains omega-three fatty acids; less than 3 grams daily is generally safe; may inhibit blood clotting; may interact with warfarin (Coumadin™)

Flaxseed oil: possibly immune-suppressing; contains omega-three and omega-six fatty acids; greater than 45 grams daily may produce diarrhea

Garlic: immune-stimulating; may inhibit blood clotting; may interact with warfarin (Coumadin™)

Ginkgo biloba: not effective for treating MS attacks; unstudied for other uses in MS; may inhibit blood clotting; may interact with warfarin (Coumadin™)

Goldenseal: possibly fatigue-producing

Grape seed extract: possibly immune-stimulating

Green tea: contains caffeine; improves mental alertness; possibly immune-stimulating; may irritate urinary tract

Guarana: contains caffeine; improves mental alertness; may irritate urinary tract

5-HTP: possible toxic effects

Kava kava: possibly effective for treating anxiety; possibly fatigue-producing

Licorice: possibly immune-stimulating; may interact with steroids; multiple possible toxic effects

Lobelia: multiple possible toxic effects

Ma huang: multiple possible toxic effects; may interact with steroids

Melatonin: possibly immune-stimulating

Niacin: see Vitamin B3

Oligomeric proanthocyanidins: possibly immune-stimulating

Passionflower: possibly fatigue-producing

Propolis: no definite therapeutic effects; unknown safety

Psyllium: FDA-approved for constipation; should not be used by people with swallowing difficulties

Pycnogenol: possibly immune-stimulating; safety of long-term use is unknown

Pyridoxine: see Vitamin B6

Royal jelly: no definite therapeutic effects; may rarely provoke asthma and cause severe allergic reactions

S-adenosylmethionine: see SAMe

Sage: possibly fatigue-producing

St. John's wort: probably effective for treating depression; possibly fatigue-producing; may interact with multiple medications, including antidepressants and antiseizure medications

SAMe: also known as S-adenosylmethionine; possibly effective for treating depression

Saw palmetto: possibly immune-stimulating

Selenium: possibly immune-stimulating; greater than 200 micrograms daily may produce multiple toxic effects

Siberian ginseng: no definite therapeutic effects; immune-stimulating; possibly fatigue-producing; may inhibit blood clotting; may interact with warfarin (Coumadin™)

Spirulina: also known as blue-green algae; contains variable amounts of gamma-linolenic acid; safety of long-term use is unknown

Stinging nettle: possibly immune-stimulating; possibly fatigue-producing; may interact with warfarin (Coumadin™)

Uva ursi: see Bearberry

Valerian: possibly effective for treating insomnia; possibly fatigue-producing; safety of long-term use is unknown

Vitamin A: chemically related to beta-carotene; immune-stimulating; greater than 15,000 IU daily may produce toxic effects; greater than 10,000 IU daily in pregnant women may produce birth defects; may increase cancer risk in smokers

Vitamin B3: also known as niacin; greater than 35 milligrams daily may produce toxic effects

Vitamin B6: also known as pyridoxine; greater than 50 milligrams daily may produce toxic effects

Vitamin B12: effective for treating documented vitamin B12 deficiency

Vitamin C: not definitely effective for treating urinary tract infections or viral infections; immune-stimulating; greater than 1,000 milligrams daily may produce toxic effects; may interact with warfarin (Coumadin™)

Vitamin D: effective for preventing and treating osteoporosis; greater than 2,000 IU daily may produce toxic effects

Vitamin E: supplements of vitamin E may be indicated with a high intake of polyunsaturated fatty acids; immune-stimulating; greater than 1,000 IU daily may produce toxic effects; may inhibit bleeding; may interact with warfarin (Coumadin™)

Vitamin K: may interact with warfarin (Coumadin™)

Yohimbe or yohimbine: multiple possible toxic effects

Zinc: possibly immune-stimulating

References

Introduction

1. Eisenberg D, Davis R, Ettner S, et al. Trends in alternative medicine use in the United States, 1990–1997. *JAMA* 1998; 280:1569–1575.
2. Eisenberg D, Kessler R, Foster C, et al. Unconventional medicine in the United States. *N Engl J Med.*1993; 328:246–252.
3. Berkman CS, Pignotti MG, Cavallo PF, et al. Use of alternative treatments by people with multiple sclerosis. *Neurorehab Neural Repair* 1999; 13:243–254.
4. Schwartz C, Laitin E, Brotman S, et al. Utilization of unconventional treatments by persons with MS: Is it alternative or complementary? *Neurology* 1999; 52:626–629.
5. Burnfield A. *Multiple Sclerosis: A Personal Exploration.* London: Souvenir Press, 1985:50.
6. Forsythe E. *Multiple Sclerosis: Exploring Sickness and Health.* London: Faber and Faber, 1988:50.
7. Winawer SJ. *Healing Lessons.* Boston: Little, Brown, 1998:28.
8. Winawer SJ. *Healing Lessons.* Boston: Little, Brown, 1998:57.

Placebos and Psychoneuroimmunology

1. Beecher HK. The powerful placebo. *JAMA* 1955; 159:1602–1606.
2. Sormani MP, Molyneaux PD, Barkhof F, et al. MRI enhancing lesion frequency from patients with MS enrolled in placebo arms of clinical trials or in natural history studies. *MRI* 1999; 17:1236–1237.
3. Hirsch RL, Johnson KP, Camenga DL. The placebo effect during a double blind trial of recombinant alpha2 interferon in multiple sclerosis patients: Immunological and clinical findings. *Neuroscience* 1988; 39:189–196.
4. Katz J. *The Silent World of Doctor and Patient.* New York: London, Collier, McMillan, 1984:191.

Acupuncture and Traditional Chinese Medicine

1. NIH Consensus Development Panel on Acupuncture. *JAMA* 1998; 280:1518–1524.
2. Spoerel WE, Paty DW, Kertesz A, et al. Acupuncture and multiple sclerosis. *CMA Journal* 1974; 110:751.
3. Smith MO, Rabinowitz N. Acupuncture treatment of multiple sclerosis: Two detailed clinical presentations. *Am J Acupuncture* 1986; 14:143–146.

4. Wang Y, Hashimoto S, Ramsum D, et al. A pilot study of the use of alternative medicine in multiple sclerosis patients with special focus on acupuncture. *Neurology* 1999; 52:A550.
5. Steinberger Antun. Specific irritability of acupuncture points as an early symptom of multiple sclerosis. *Am J Chinese Med* 1986; 14:175–178.
6. Yi S, Xiaoyan L. A review on traditional Chinese medicine in prevention and treatment of multiple sclerosis. *J Trad Chinese Med* 1999;19:65–73.

Bee Venom Therapy and Other Forms of Apitherapy

1. Lublin FD, Oshinsky RJ, Perreault, M, et al. Effect of honey bee venom on EAE. *Neurology* 1998; 50:A424.

Cooling Therapy

1. Capell E, Gardella M, Leandri M, et al. Lowering body temperature with a cooling suit as symptomatic treatment for thermosensitive multiple sclerosis patients. *Ital J Neurol Sci* 1995; 16:533–539.
2. Flensner G, Lindencrona C. The cooling-suit: A study of ten multiple sclerosis patients' experience in daily life. *J Adv Nurs* 1999; 29:1444–1453.

Craniosacral Therapy

1. Greenman PE, McPartland JM. Cranial findings and iatrogenesis from craniosacral manipulation in patients with traumatic brain syndrome. *J Am Osteopath Assoc* 1995; 95:182–188,191–192.

Diets and Fatty Acid Supplements

1. Swank RL. Multiple sclerosis: Twenty years on low fat diet. *Arch Neurol* 1970; 23:460–474.
2. Swank RL, Dugan BB. Effect of low saturated fat diet in early and late cases of multiple sclerosis. *Lancet* 1990; 336:37–39.
3. Miller JHD, Zilkha KJ, Langman MJS, et al. Double-blind trial of linoleate supplementation of the diet in multiple sclerosis. *Br Med J* 1973; 1:765–768.
4. Bates D, Fawcett PRW, Shaw DA, et al. Polyunsaturated fatty acids in treatment of acute remitting multiple sclerosis. *Br Med J* 1978; 2:1390–1391.
5. Paty DW, Cousin HK, Read S, et al. Linoleic acid in multiple sclerosis: Failure to show any therapeutic benefit. *Acta Neurol Scand* 1978; 58:53–58.
6. Dworkin RH, Bates D, Millar JHD, et al. Linoleic acid and multiple sclerosis: A reanalysis of three double-blind trials. *Neurology* 1984; 34:1441–1445.
7. Bates D, Fawcett PRW, Shaw DA, et al. Trial of polyunsaturated fatty acids in non-relapsing multiple sclerosis. *Br Med J*, 1977; 10:932–933.
8. Gibson Robert A, Lines David R, Neumann Mark A. Gamma linolenic acid (GLA) content of encapsulated evening primrose oil products. *Lipids* 1992: 27:82–84.
9. Bates D, Cartlidge NEF, French JM, et al. A double-blind controlled trial of long chain n-3 polyunsaturated fatty acids in the treatment of multiple sclerosis. *J Neurol Neurosurg Psychiatry* 1989; 52:18–22.

10. Goldberg P, Fleming MC, Picard EH. Multiple sclerosis: Decreased relapse rate through dietary supplementation with calcium, magnesium and vitamin D. *Med Hypoth* 1986; 21:193–200.
11. Rowland L (ed.). *Merritt's Textbook of Neurology.* Baltimore: Williams & Wilkins, 1995:824.
12. Paty DW, Ebers GC (eds.). *Multiple Sclerosis.* Philadelphia: FA Davis, 1998:510.
13. Kesselring J. *Multiple Sclerosis.* New York: Cambridge University Press, 1997:203.
14. Bates D. Lipids and multiple sclerosis. *Biochem Soc Trans* 1989; 17:289–291.

Exercise

1.   Petajan JH, Gappmaier E, White AT, et al. Impact of aerobic training on fitness and quality of life in multiple sclerosis. *Ann Neurol* 1996; 39:432–441.

Feldenkrais

1.   Johnson SK, Frederick J, Kaufman M, et al. A controlled investigation of bodywork in multiple sclerosis. *J Alt Complem Med* 1999; 5:237–243.

Herbs

1.   Korwin-Piotrowska T, Nocon D, Stankowska-Chomicz A, et al. Experience of padma 28 in multiple sclerosis. *Phytother Res* 1992; 6:133–136.
2.   Blumenthal M (ed.). *The Complete German Commission E Monographs: Therapeutic Guide to Herbal Medicines.* Austin: American Botanical Council, 1998:441.
3.   Brinker F. Herb *Contraindications and Drug Interactions.* Oregon: Eclectic Medical Publishers, 1998:150–151.

Hippotherapy and Therapeutic Horseback Riding

1.   MacKay-Lyons M, Conway C, Roberts W. Effects of therapeutic riding on patients with multiple sclerosis: A preliminary trial. *Proceedings of the 6th International Therapeutic Riding Congress* 1998; 8:173–178.
2.   Pfotenhauer M, Leyerer U, David E, et al. Hippotherapy, scientific program in Herdecke, an example. *Proceedings of the 7th International Therapeutic Riding Congress* 1991; August:46–57.

Homeopathy

1.   Swayne J. *Homeopathic Method: Implications for Clinical Practice and Medical Science.* New York: Churchill Livingstone, 1998:191.
2.   Kleijnen J, Knipschild P, ter Riet G. Clinical trials of homoeopathy. *Br Med J* 1991; 302:316–326.
3.   Linde K, Clausius N, Ramirez G, et al. Are the clinical effects of homoeopathy placebo effects? A meta-analysis of placebo-controlled trails. *Lancet* 1997; 350:834–843.

Hyperbaric Oxygen

1. Fischer BH, Marks M, Reich T. Hyperbaric oxygen treatment of multiple sclerosis. A randomized, placebo-controlled, double-blind study. *N Engl J Med* 1983; 308:181–186.
2. Kleijnen J, Knipschild P. Hyperbaric oxygen for multiple sclerosis: Review of controlled trials. *Acta Neurol Scand* 1995; 91:330–334.

Hypnosis and Guided Imagery

1. Maguire BL. The effects of imagery on attitudes and moods in multiple sclerosis patients. *Alt Ther* 1996; 2:75–79.
2. Hall H, Minnes L, Olness K. The psychophysiology of voluntary immunomodulation. *Int J Neurosci* 1993; 69:221–234.

Magnets and Electromagnetic Therapy

1. Guseo A. Pulsing electromagnetic field therapy of multiple sclerosis by the Gyuling-Bordás device: Double-blind, cross-over and open studies. *J Bioelec* 1987; 6:23–35.
2. Nielsen JF, Sinkjaer T, Jakobsen J. Treatment of spasticity with repetitive magnetic stimulation: A double-blind placebo-controlled study. *Multiple Sclerosis* 1996; 2:227–232.
3. Richards TL, Lappin MS, Acosta-Urquidi J, et al. Double-blind study of pulsing magnetic field effects on multiple sclerosis. *J Alt Complem Med* 1997; 3:21–29.

Marijuana

1. Schon F, Hart PE, Hodgson TL, et al. Suppression of pendular nystagmus by smoking cannabis in a patient with multiple sclerosis. *Neurology* 1999; 53:2209–2210.
2. Consroe P, Musty R, Rein J, et al. The perceived effects of smoked cannabis on patients with multiple sclerosis. *Eur Neurol* 1997; 38:44–48.
3. Baker D, Pryce G, Croxford J, et al. Cannabinoids control spasticity and tremor in a multiple sclerosis model. *Nature* 2000; 404:84–87.

Massage

1. Hernandez-Reif M, Field T, Field T, et al. Multiple sclerosis patients benefit from massage therapy. *J Bodywork Movement Ther* 1998; 2:168–174.
2. Forsythe E. *Multiple Sclerosis: Exploring Sickness and Health.* London: Faber and Faber, 1988:129.

Meditation

1. Mandel Allan R, Keller Sandra M. Stress management in rehabilitation. *Arch Phys Med Rehabil* 1986; 67:375–379.
2. Smith GR, McKenzie JM, Marmer DJ, et al. Psychologic modulation of the human immune response to Varicella Zoster. *Arch Intern Med* 1985; 145: 2110–2112.

Pets

1. Dossey L. The healing power of pets: A look at animal-assisted therapy. *Alt Ther* 1997; 3:8–16.

The Pilates Method and The Physical Mind Method

1. Hutchinson MR, Tremain L, Christiansen J, et al. Improving leaping ability in elite rhythmic gymnasts. *Med Science Sports Ex* 1998; 30:1543–1547.

Prayer and Spirituality

1. Bryd RC. Positive therapeutic effects of intercessory prayer in a coronary care unit population. *South Med J* 1988; 81:826–829.
2. Harris WS, Gowda M, Kolb J, et al. A randomized, controlled trial of the effects of remote, intercessory prayer on outcomes in patients admitted to the coronary care unit. *Arch Intern Med* 1999; 159:2273–2278.

Procarin

1. Gillson G, Wright JV, Ballasiotes G. Transdermal histamine in multiple sclerosis. Part 1: Clinical experience. *Alt Med Rev* 1999; 4:424–428.

T'ai Chi

1. Husted C, Pham L, Hekking A, et al. Improving quality of life for people with chronic conditions: The example of t'ai chi and multiple sclerosis. *Alt Ther* 1999; 5:70–74.

Therapeutic Touch

1. Rosa L, Rosa E, Sarner L, et al. A close look at therapeutic touch. *JAMA* 1998; 279:1005–1010.
2. Long R, Bernhardt P, Evans W. Perception of conventional sensory cues as an alternative to the postulated 'human energy field' of therapeutic touch. *Sci Rev Alt Med* 1999; 3:53–61.

Toxins

1. Ames BN, Magaw R, Gold LS. Ranking possible carcinogenic hazards. *Science* 1987; 236:271–280.

Tragerwork

1. Witt PL, MacKinnon J. Trager psychophysical integration. A method to improve chest mobility of patients with chronic lung disease. *Phys Ther* 1986; 66:214–217.

Vitamins, Minerals, and Other Nonherbal Supplements

1. Mai J, Sorensen PS, Hansen JC. High dose antioxidant supplementation to MS patients. *Biol Trace Elem Res* 1990; 24:109–117.
2. Goldberg P, Fleming MC, Picard EH. Multiple sclerosis: Decreased relapse rate through dietary supplementation with calcium, magnesium and vitamin D. *Med Hypoth* 1986; 21:193–200.
3. Fleming John O, Hummel Ann L, Beinlich Brad R, et al. Vitamin D treatment of relapsing-remitting multiple sclerosis (RRMS): A MRI-based pilot study. *Neurology* 2000; 54:A338.

Index

Demos Medical Publishing, Inc. publishes numerous books on multiple sclerosis. These include:

Meeting the Challenge of Progressive Multiple Sclerosis
Patricia K. Coyle and June Halper

Multiple Sclerosis: A Guide for the Newly Diagnosed
Nancy J. Holland, T. Jock Murray, and Stephen C. Reingold

Multiple Sclerosis: The Questions You Have—The Answers You Need,
2nd edition
Rosalind C. Kalb

Multiple Sclerosis: A Guide for Families
Rosalind C. Kalb

Multiple Sclerosis: Your Legal Rights, 2nd edition
Lanny E. Perkins and Sara D. Perkins

300 Tips for Making Life with Multiple Sclerosis Easier
Shelley Peterman Schwarz

Multiple Sclerosis: The Guide to Treatment and Management, 5th edition
Chris H. Polman, Alan J. Thompson,
T. Jock Murray, and W. Ian McDonald

Employment Issues in Multiple Sclerosis
Phillip D. Rumrill, Jr.

Symptom Management in Multiple Sclerosis, 3rd edition
Randall T. Schapiro

To receive additional information on these or any of our other titles,
call our toll-free number:
(800) 532-8663

Demos Medical Publishing, Inc.
386 Park Avenue South
New York, NY 10016
Phone (212) 683-0072
Fax (212) 683-0118
E-mail: orderdept@demospub.com
Website: demosmedpub.com